RESISTANCE BAND
WORKOUT
FOR SENIORS

Fully **Illustrated Workout Plan** for Reclaiming **Strength**, Enhancing **Flexibility**, and Achieving **Weight Loss** in **Just 28 Days**

FitLife Solutions – Grow Your Health

Explore More from Fitlife Solution

Browse our collection today and take the first step towards a healthier, fitter you!

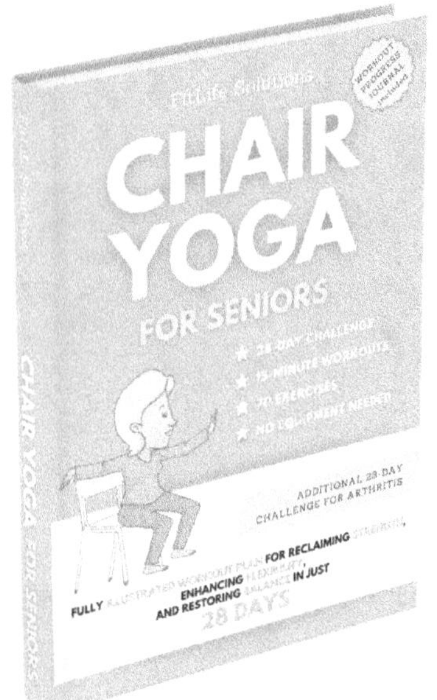

CHAIR YOGA FOR SENIORS:

Fully Illustrated Workout Plan for Reclaiming Strength, Enhancing Flexibility, and Restoring Balance in Just 28 Days

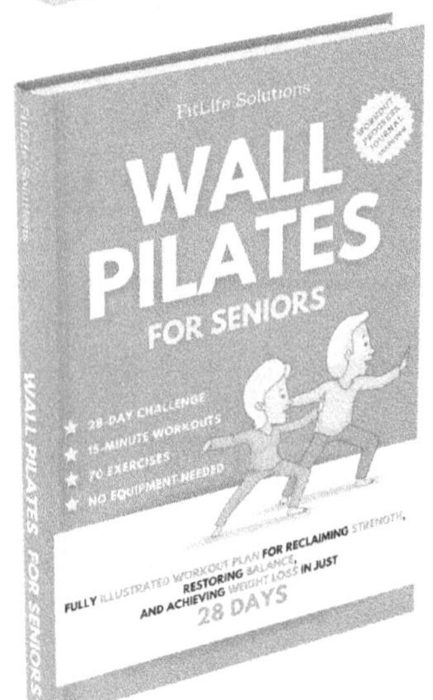

WALL PILATES FOR SENIORS:

Fully Illustrated Workout Plan for Reclaiming Strength, Restoring Balance, and Achieving Weight Loss in Just 28 Days

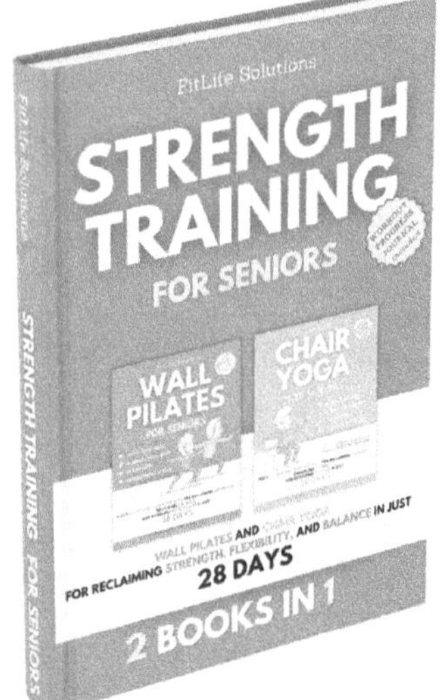

STRENGTH TRAINING FOR SENIORS:

2 Books in 1
Wall Pilates and Chair Yoga for Reclaiming Strength, Flexibility, and Balance in Just 28 Days

Table of Contents

About the Author

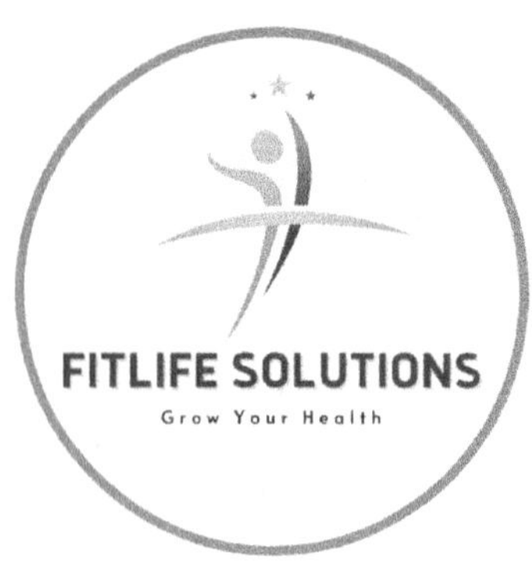

FitLife Solutions is a leading provider of fitness programs tailored to individuals of all ages and diverse needs. Our mission is to empower people to live healthier, happier lives through personalized fitness solutions.

At FitLife Solutions, we understand unique fitness goals and requirements and, therefore, offer a wide range of programs designed to cater to the specific needs of each individual. Whether you're a busy professional looking for more efficient workouts, an individual who has specialized fitness needs, or a senior wanting to improve flexibility and mobility, there's a program just for you.

Our team of certified trainers and experienced fitness experts work effortlessly to develop innovative, effective workout plans for the highest level of effectiveness, safety, and enjoyment. The latest research in exercise science is combined with practical, real-world applications when we create programs that deliver tangible results.

At FitLife Solutions, we strongly believe fitness is for everyone, regardless of ability, age, or background. We make fitness accessible, enjoyable, and rewarding for everyone, and we support you along your journey to better health and wellness.

Introduction

Welcome to the transformative world of resistance band training designed specifically for seniors. This book takes you on a journey to experience the rejuvenating power of exercise using resistance bands, a versatile and effective tool for maintaining physical health and vitality. Resistance band training offers a comprehensive solution to help with joint stiffness and increase flexibility and strength. This program is designed to be adaptable, allowing you to adjust the intensity of the exercises to match your fitness level and goals. The simplicity and effectiveness of resistance band training make it an ideal choice for seniors seeking to maintain an active and healthy lifestyle. With resistance bands, you can achieve a comprehensive workout without the need for heavy and expensive equipment or a gym membership, making it an accessible option for everyone.

A 28-day workout plan is outlined in this book. Your life will be changed by spending 15 minutes each day. The exercises were carefully selected to be manageable and challenging enough to move through at your own pace and see results. The range of exercises focuses on different muscle groups and gentle stretches to maximize your health and vitality.

So, are you ready? Let's get started on this path toward good health and well-being. Just add your commitment and consistency to reap the benefits of resistance band training. You can enjoy a better, more energetic life. Let's get started!

Happy training,
FitLife Solutions Team

Special Bonus Offer!

Hello Readers,

You are a valued member of our fitness community, so we're excited to offer a wonderful bonus to help you on your path to fitness! Simply scan the **QR code** or **click on the link below**, and you'll be directed to our supplementary **Workout Progress Journal**.

QR code:

or **link:** <u>Workout Progress Journal</u>

The journal will assist you along your way toward fitness by providing a means to track your workouts, set individual goals, and monitor the progress you are making. The easy-to-use format and comprehensively-designed journal is a great tool to keep you on track, motivated, and accountable as you reach your fitness goals.

Don't miss out on this incredible opportunity to take your fitness journey to the next level.

Happy training,
FitLife Solutions Team

What is Resistance Band Training

Resistance band training is a form of strength training that uses elastic bands to provide resistance against muscle contractions. This type of training is versatile, portable, and effective for people of all fitness levels.

What are the basic principles of resistance band training?

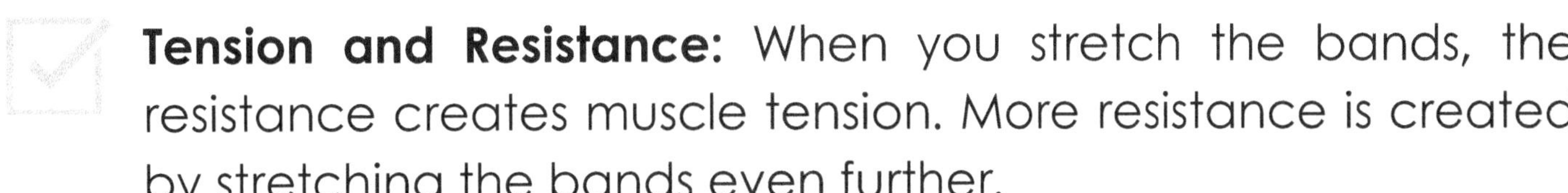

Tension and Resistance: When you stretch the bands, the resistance creates muscle tension. More resistance is created by stretching the bands even further.

Variable Resistance: Unlike free weights, which provide constant resistance, the resistance from bands increases as they are stretched, offering variable resistance throughout the range of motion.

Progressive Overload: By using thicker bands, combining them, and adding to the number of repetitions and sets, you can increase resistance.

Resistance band training is an effective and accessible way to improve strength, flexibility, and overall fitness. Whether you're a beginner or an experienced athlete, incorporating resistance bands into your workout routine can offer a diverse range of exercises and benefits.

Selecting the Right Resistance Band

To have a safe and effective workout, especially for seniors, it's important to select the appropriate resistance band. These guidelines should help you choose the best band for your training.

TYPES OF RESISTANCE BANDS

We use two different kinds of resistance bands for our workout program.

- **Loop Bands:** Loop bands are elastic bands that form a closed loop. They are also called mini bands or resistance loop bands and are used in a variety of exercises, including upper body, lower body, and core workouts. They are used frequently for squats, leg lifts, lunges, shoulder lateral raises, hip abduction, and arm curls. Loop bands are especially useful for working the shoulders, thighs, glutes, and hips.

- **Therapy Bands:** Therapy bands are long flat strips of elastic material. They are also known as physical therapy bands or flat resistance bands. Typically, they are used in physical therapy and rehabilitation settings to help with rehabilitation exercises, flexibility, and muscle strengthening. The bands help improve joint mobility, resistance training, and stretching. Some specific exercises to do with therapy bands include abdominal crunches, leg lifts, chest presses, bicep curls, and tricep extensions. A versatile tool, exercises with bands can target the upper body, lower body, and core muscle groups.

Selecting the Right Resistance Band

RESISTANCE LEVEL

The different colored resistance bands have various levels of resistance. A common color-coding classification is used for the bands:

- **Yellow (Light):** Appropriate for those recovering from injuries and also beginners, they provide the lightest resistance.

- **Green (Medium):** Appropriate for intermediate users, they provide moderate resistance to increase strength and endurance.

- **Red (Heavy):** Appropriate for advanced users and those who want a more intensive workout, they provide a higher level of resistance.

- **Black (Ultra Heavy):** Appropriate for the most experienced individuals and athletes, they provide the highest level of resistance.

When selecting resistance bands, it's suggested to begin with a lighter resistance. Then as your strength increases, move toward a higher level. Note, that the resistance band levels can vary among brands. So, it's important to look at the manufacturer's specifications. There may be additional colors available besides the standard colors described above. For example, there could be an extra light option (gray) and an extra heavy option (purple).

Resistance Band Training Benefits for Seniors

Resistance band training offers numerous benefits, making it an excellent choice for seniors looking to maintain their fitness and improve their overall health. Let's look at some important advantages:

 **Versatile:** A variety of exercises can be performed with bands to focus on different muscle groups. This helps you enjoy a comprehensive workout that fits your needs.

 **Cost-Effective:** The bands are affordable especially compared to other gym equipment so you can have an effective workout and not spend a lot of money.

 **Adjustable Resistance:** The level of resistance can be modified easily to best match your fitness level and goals. As you exercise more and your body gets stronger, you can combine bands or use thicker ones to continue to strengthen the muscles and make fitness gains.

 **Joint-Friendly:** Offering a low-impact form of exercise, resistance bands reduce the risk of injury. They are a perfect choice for those with joint issues or others recovering from injury.

 **Improves Flexibility and Strength:** Through regular use, the bands can help seniors enhance flexibility, build muscle strength, and improve overall mobility, enabling a more active, independent lifestyle.

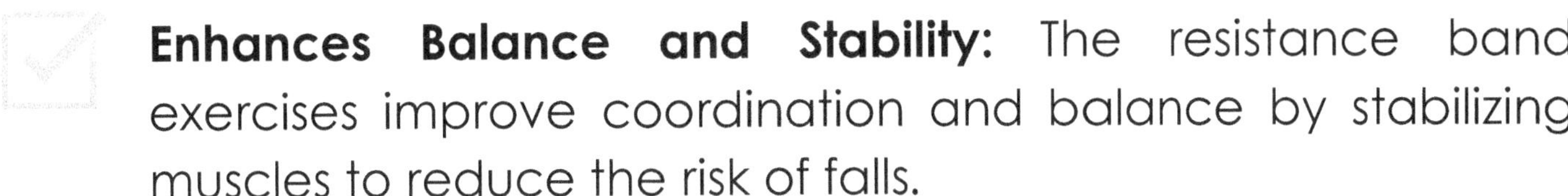

Enhances Balance and Stability: The resistance band exercises improve coordination and balance by stabilizing muscles to reduce the risk of falls.

Exercise Variety: Resistance bands are a versatile tool for working out. They meet many fitness needs including stretching, strength training, mobility exercises, and rehabilitation.

Rehabilitation and Recovery: Commonly used in physical therapy and rehabilitation, resistance bands help with injury recovery and improve muscle function. This makes them a great tool for those experiencing chronic conditions or recovering from surgeries.

Portable: The lightweight compact bands can be taken with you and stored easily. That makes them a great fit for working out at home or away.

By adding resistance band training to a senior's fitness routine, improvements can be made in flexibility, balance, strength, and overall health. Resistance bands are an invaluable addition to any exercise program.

Safety Tips and Precautions for Resistance Band Training

Like other types of exercise, safety tips and precautions should be followed. This helps prevent injury and allows for a safe, successful workout. Keep these important points in mind:

- **Consult a Healthcare Professional:** Talk to your healthcare provider before beginning any new exercise program. This is especially important if you have any pre-existing health condition or injury.

- **Inspect the Bands Regularly:** Always inspect your resistance bands before using them for any signs of damage, wear, or tear. Look for holes, frays, and cracks that could lead the band to snap. If you see any damage, replace the resistance band to prevent an accident.

- **Use the Right Resistance Level:** Always start with a lighter resistance band and then you can increase the resistance gradually as you continue to build strength. This is especially important if you are new to this type of training. Don't overstretch the bands (they have an intended length); they can lose elasticity and even break.

- **Warm-Up and Cool-Down Periods:** Beginning each workout with a warm-up period is necessary to ready your muscles and joints for exercise. A proper warm-up helps improve your performance and prevents injuries along the way. After your workout, take time to cool down and stretch. Your muscles will thank you for giving them time to recover and reduce soreness.

Safety Tips and Precautions for Resistance Band Training

- **Focus on Controlled Movements and the Proper Technique:** Executing the correct form for each exercise helps to maximize its effectiveness and minimize injury. Every exercise needs to be done with slow, controlled movements. Don't snap or jerk the resistance band to cause potential injury.

- **Positioning and Grip:** It's necessary to hold the bands firmly and with a proper grip. When using loop bands, make sure they are correctly positioned on your body so they don't slip.

- **Always Listen to Your Body:** Try to differentiate between persistent pain from a challenging workout or the normal discomfort from an exercise. Give yourself enough time to rest and recover between the workouts so you don't overtrain and cause injury.

These safety tips and precautions will help you enjoy and maximize the benefits of resistance band training and minimize the risk of any injury. They will also help to ensure a safe and effective workout. Safety is a top priority so listen to your body throughout the workout sessions.

Breathing

Proper breathing techniques are essential in resistance band training to maximize performance, improve oxygen delivery to muscles, and ensure safety. Let's look at incorporating effective breathing into the workouts:

1. THE BASIC BREATHING TECHNIQUE

- **Inhale Before the Effort:** Take a deep breath through your nose before beginning the exercise's exertion phase to prepare your body and provide stability.

- **Exhale During the Effort:** Exhale steadily and slowly through your mouth during the exercise's exertion phase (when performing the movement against resistance) to help generate force and maintain control.

- **Inhale During the Return:** As you return to the starting position, inhale again as you prepare for the next repetition.

2. PROPER BREATHING MATTERS

- **Oxygen Supply:** By breathing properly, your muscles get sufficient oxygen, which enhances endurance and performance.

- **Core Stability:** With coordinated breathing, the diaphragm and core muscles are engaged, reducing the risk of injury and providing stability.

Breathing

- **Blood Pressure Regulation:** Exhale during exertion to prevent excessive increases in blood pressure. This helps promote cardiovascular safety.

- **Focus and Relaxation:** Controlled breathing helps with mental focus and reduces stress, allowing more effective and enjoyable workouts.

3. PACED BREATHING

- **Match Breath with Movement:** Coordinate your breathing rhythm as you exercise (take longer and deeper breaths for slower movements and breathe more rapidly yet controlled for quicker movements).

- **Avoid Holding Breath:** During exertion, don't hold your breath (i.e., the Valsalva maneuver); it can contribute to a spike in blood pressure and reduce oxygen flow.

4. DIAPHRAGMATIC BREATHING

- **Deep Belly Breathing:** Rather than focus on shallow breaths into your chest, focus on breathing deeply into your diaphragm to maximize lung capacity and oxygen intake.

Incorporating proper breathing techniques into resistance band training will enhance your workout efficiency. This, in turn, will help support your cardiovascular health and you will attain better overall results.

What is needed for Resistance Band Training

There is minimal equipment required for resistance band training. Essential items to get you started include:

- ☑ **Resistance bands:** Look for loop bands and therapy bands with the appropriate resistance levels.

- ☑ **Exercise mat:** A nonslip exercise mat provides adequate support and cushioning for floor exercises.

- ☑ **Sturdy chair:** A stable and sturdy chair with a straight back and without arms or supportive armrests is ideal. Don't use a chair with wheels, legs that can easily slide on the floor, or one that is too soft or unstable.

- ☑ **Stopwatch or Timer:** Use a stopwatch or timer to track the duration of exercise and rest periods to ensure you stay on schedule.

- ☑ **Comfortable clothing:** Your clothing should be stretchable and breathable to move freely.

- ☑ **Water bottle:** To stay hydrated throughout the workout, keep a water bottle nearby filled with water.

- ☑ **Towel:** A towel is helpful to wipe away any sweat and keep your comfort level high as you complete the workout.

What is needed for Resistance Band Training

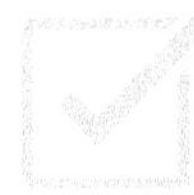 **Workout space:** You need ample space to perform the exercises safely without bumping into furniture or other things.

 **Positive mindset:** Your attitude and willingness to challenge yourself go a long way to increase the benefits of your exercise. Always be open to adapting the exercises to your fitness level and ability. Listen to your body to best match the exercise sessions to your needs.

By having these essential items, you will be ready for productive and enjoyable resistance band training.

Types of Exercises: Warm-Ups

Head Circles (Right, Left)

This is a perfect exercise for those who want to stretch their shoulders and release tension from the neck. (You can reduce discomfort and decrease your risk of injury by improving your neck flexibility).

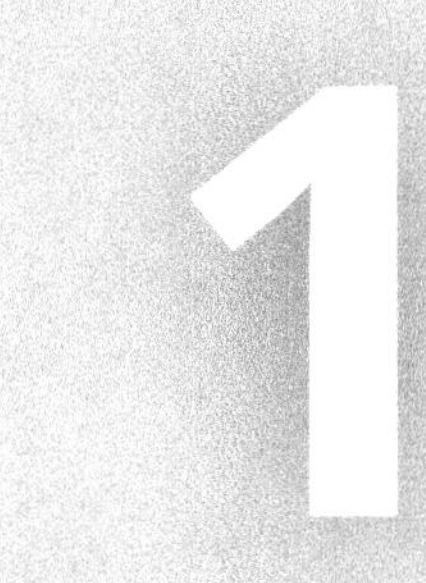

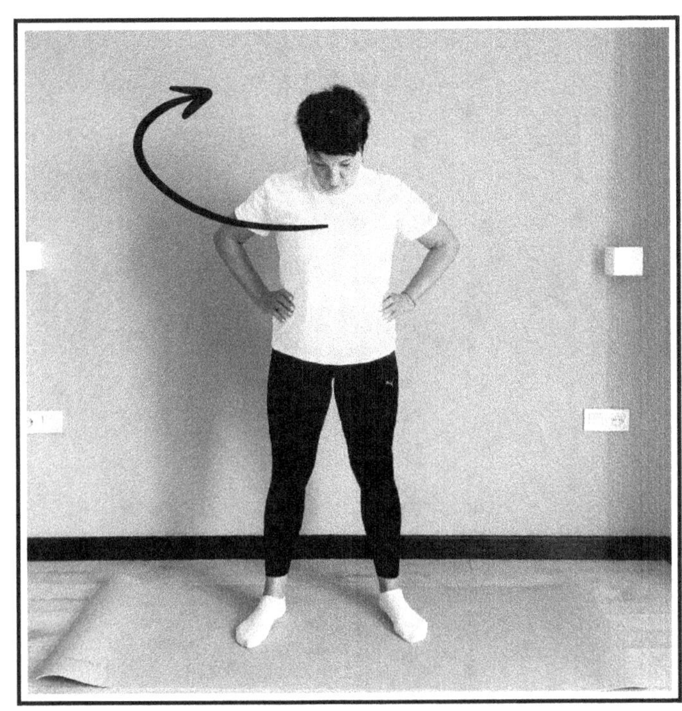

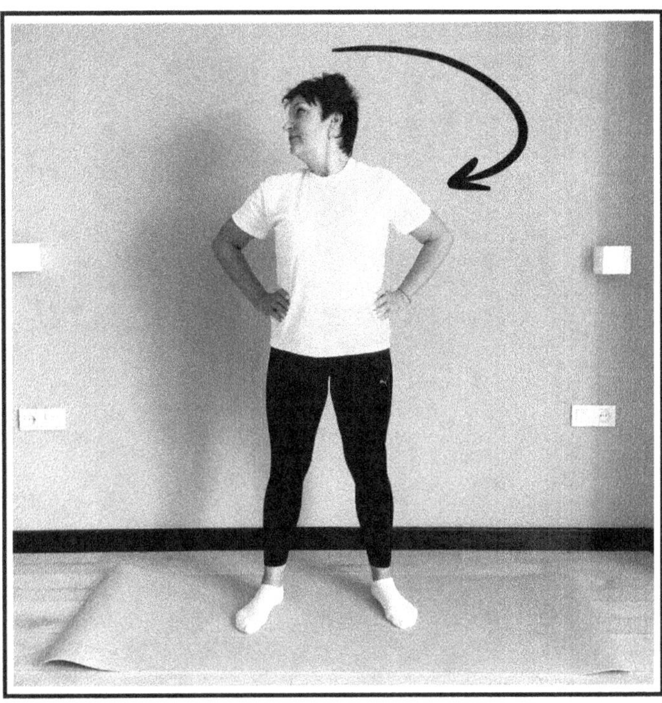

PROCEDURE:

1. Face forward
2. Slowly tilt your head forward; start rolling it to the right, then back, and to the left
3. Gently roll your head to the front
4. Repeat the movement
5. Perform the exercise on the left side

SUGGESTED TIPS:

- Don't rush through the exercise; move your head in slow, gentle circles
- Relax your shoulders
- Keep the movements fluid
- Avoid this exercise or be careful if you are suffering from disc problems, post-fracture, or whiplash

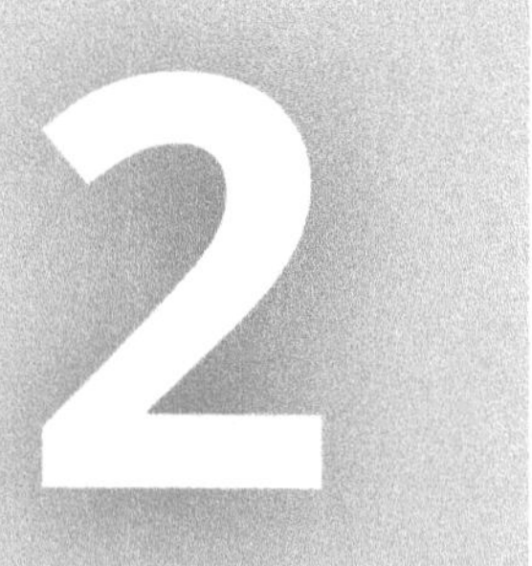

Shoulder Circles
(Forward, Backward)

Shoulder circles are a perfect warm-up exercise that activates the shoulder joints before working out. This exercise also improves mobility and helps reduce shoulder pain.

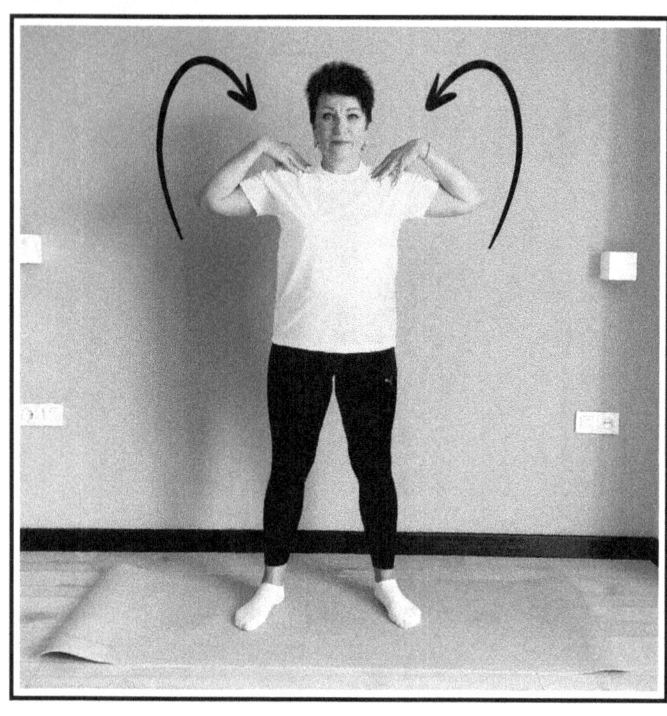

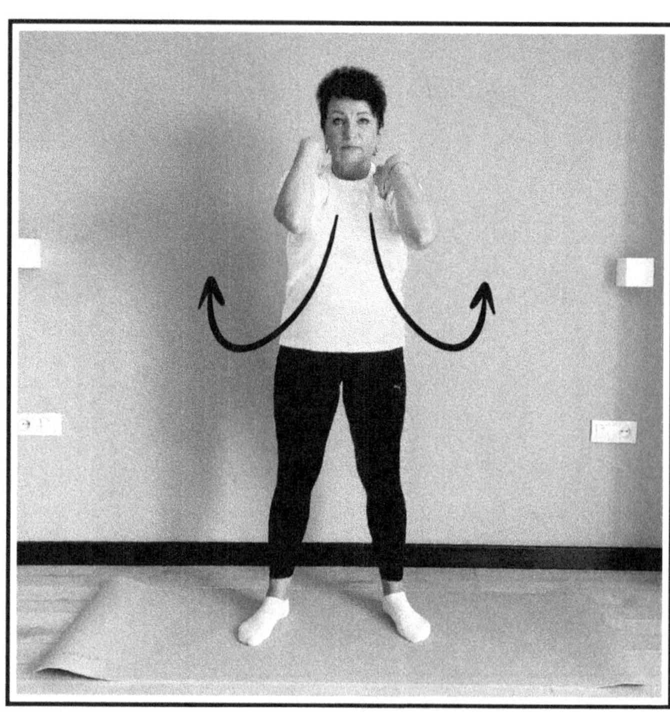

PROCEDURE:

1. Place your fingertips on your shoulders while in a standing position
2. Circle your shoulders forward
3. Repeat the movement
4. Perform the exercise by moving your shoulders backward

SUGGESTED TIPS:

- Don't go too fast
- Keep your body relaxed with your motions controlled and slow; look straight ahead

Arm Rotations
(Forward, Backward)

This is a great warm-up exercise to get your shoulders ready to go!

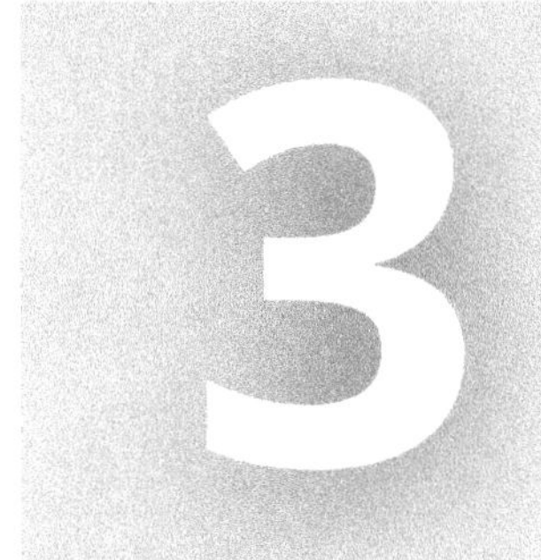

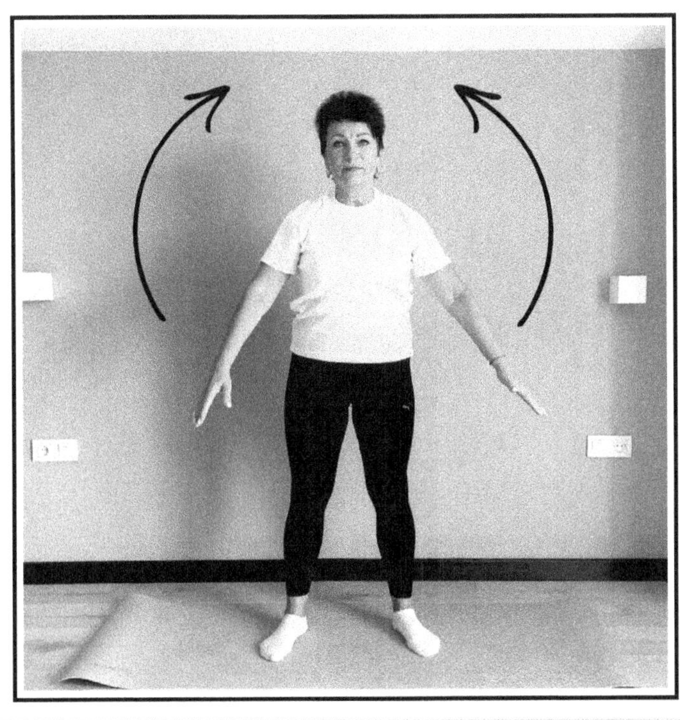

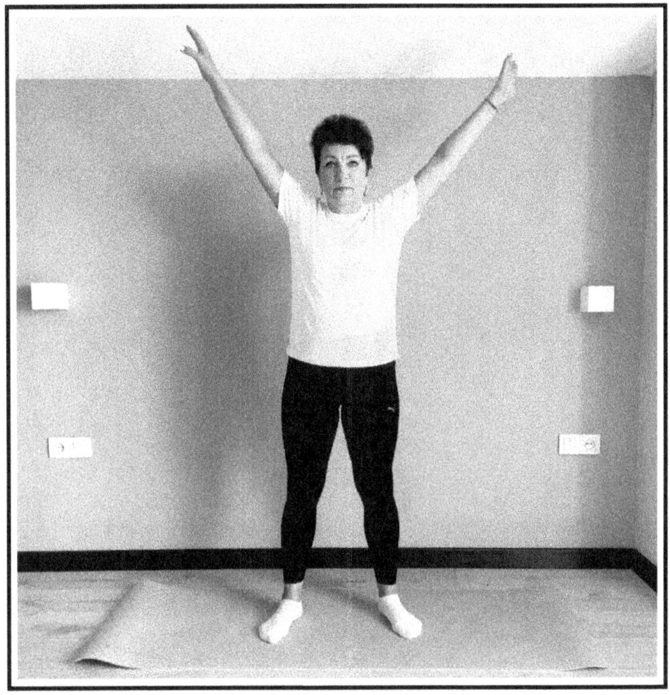

1. Stand tall with your hands on the sides
2. Swing your arms forward in large circles
3. Repeat the movement
4. Perform the exercise by swinging your arms backward

- Maximize the range of motion (it's easier to circle your arms forward but try to do so when reaching backward, too)
- Start slowly while extending your arms and then speed up as the shoulders warm-up

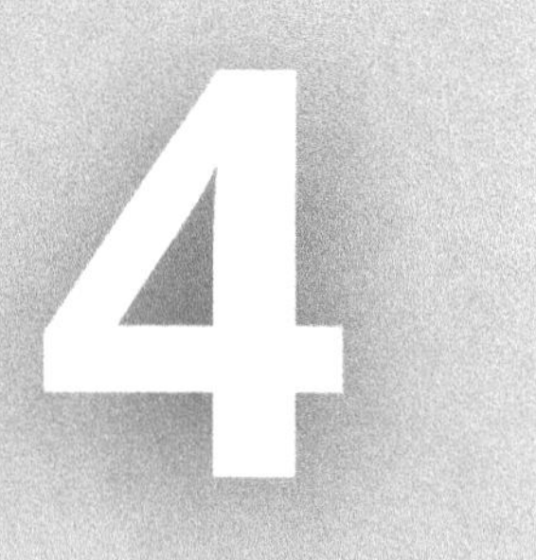

4 Elbow Rotations
(Outward/Inward)

This elbow rotation is a fun warm-up that will get your arms moving.

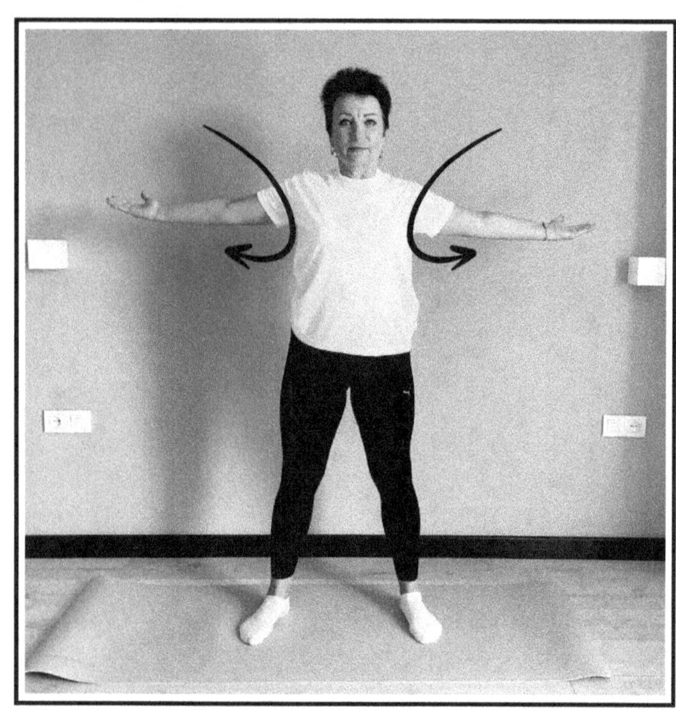 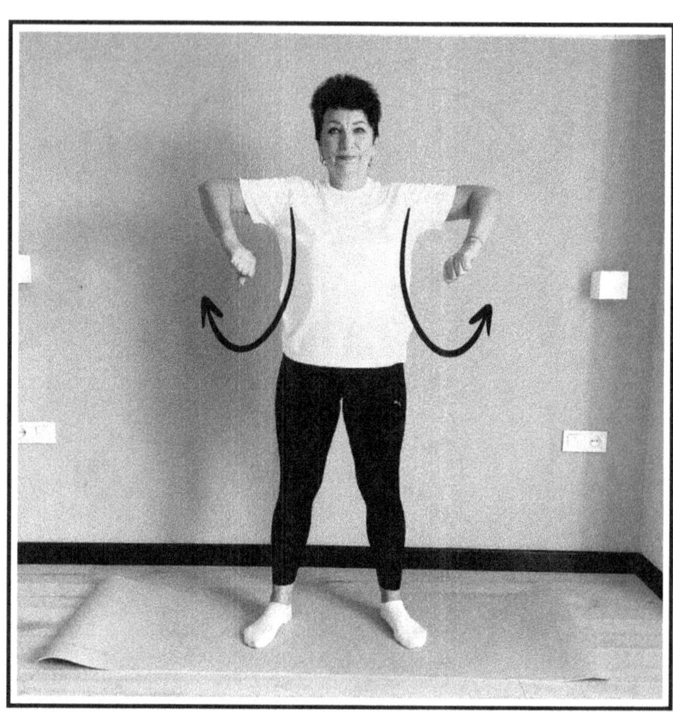

PROCEDURE:

1. Stand tall and hold your arms out to the sides as you keep your elbows even with your shoulders
2. Swing your forearms up toward your head to start, eventually completing a full outward circle
3. Repeat the movement
4. Perform the exercise swinging your forearm in toward your ribs to start eventually completing an inward circle

SUGGESTED TIPS:

- Don't go too fast too soon (have the motion down first, then speed up)
- Try to keep the elbows steady while swinging your arms

Hula Rotations
(Clockwise/Counter-Clockwise)

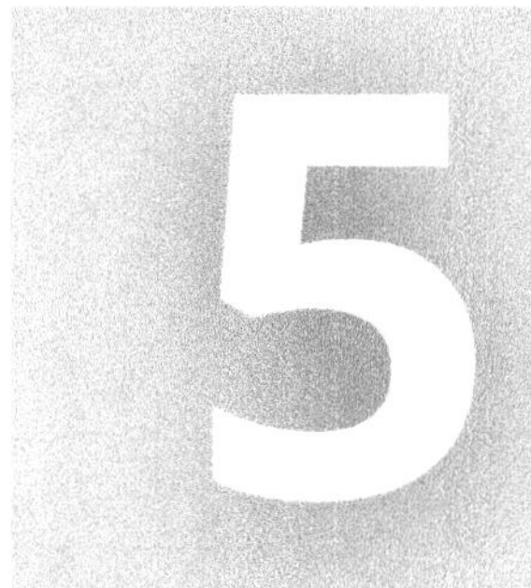

This fun motion is an easy warm-up to loosen the joints and get the blood flowing.

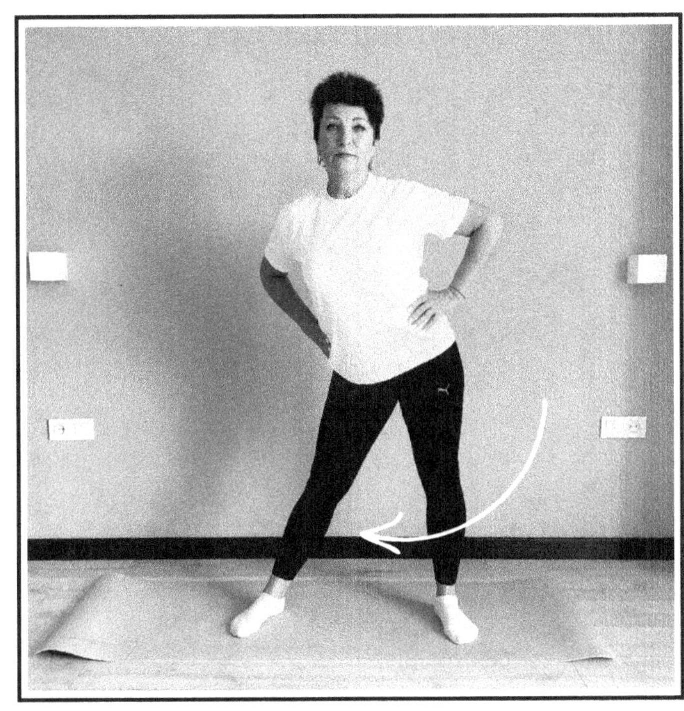

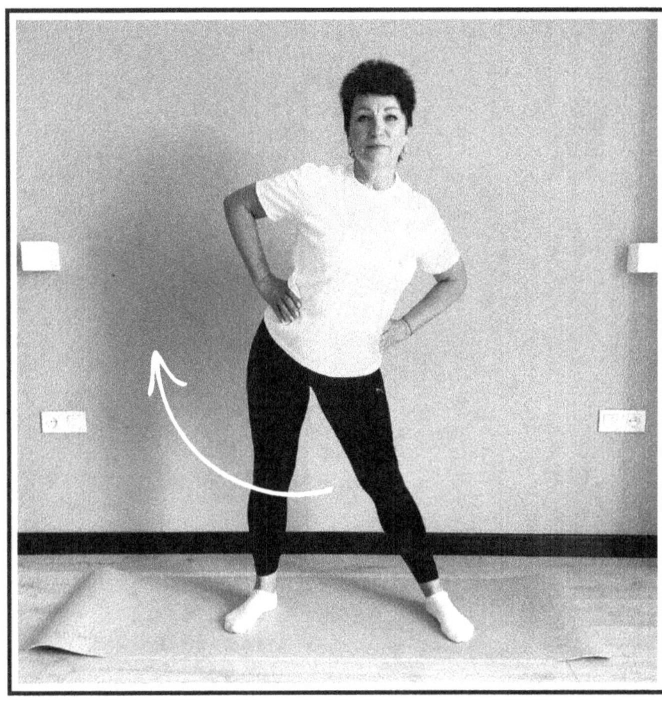

1. Stand upright with your hands on the hips
2. Move your hips in a circle in a clockwise direction as if you were hula-hooping
3. Repeat the movement
4. Perform the exercise in a counter-clockwise direction

- Don't bend at the waist but try to make a continuous motion to get your hips moving
- Let your hips loosen up

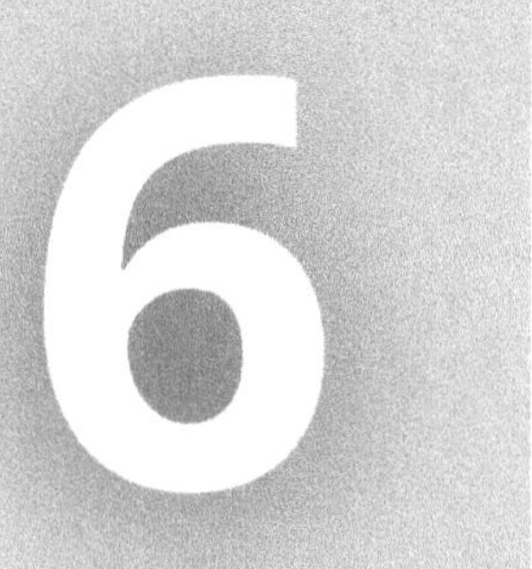

Knee Rotations
(Clockwise/Counter-Clockwise)

This exercise is a great warm-up to get your knees loosened up and ready to go!

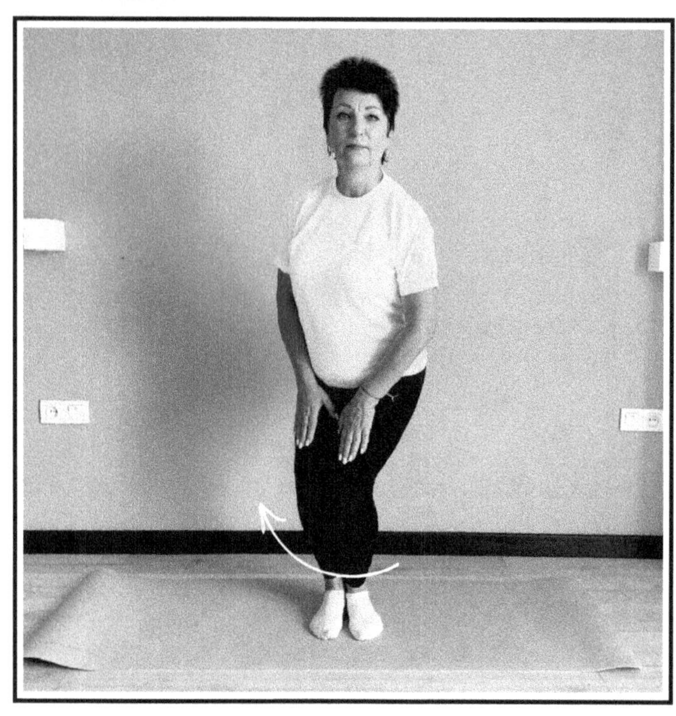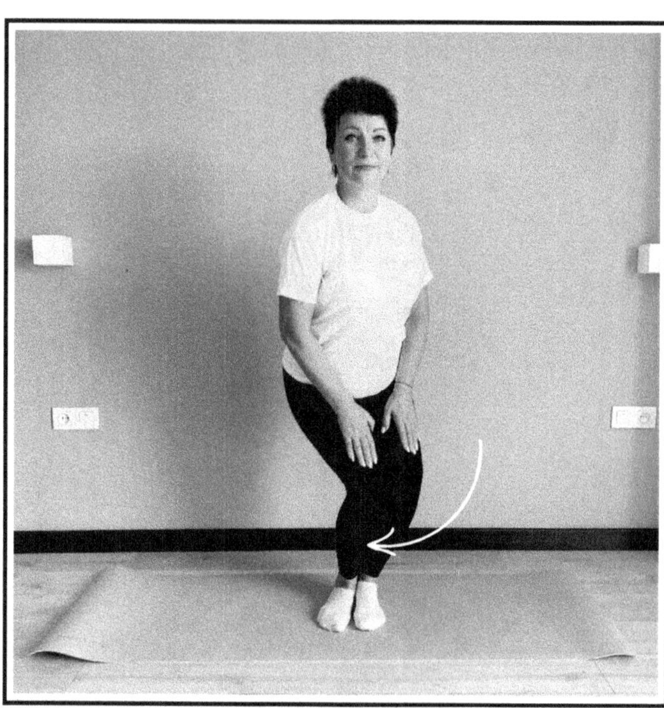

PROCEDURE:

1. Stand and put your hands on your knees
2. Move your knees clockwise in a circular motion
3. Repeat the exercise counterclockwise

SUGGESTED TIPS:

- Keep your knees and feet together
- Relax your legs

PAGE 24

Wide Leg Good Morning

7

The Romanian deadlift (RDL) version will lift and tone your glutes.

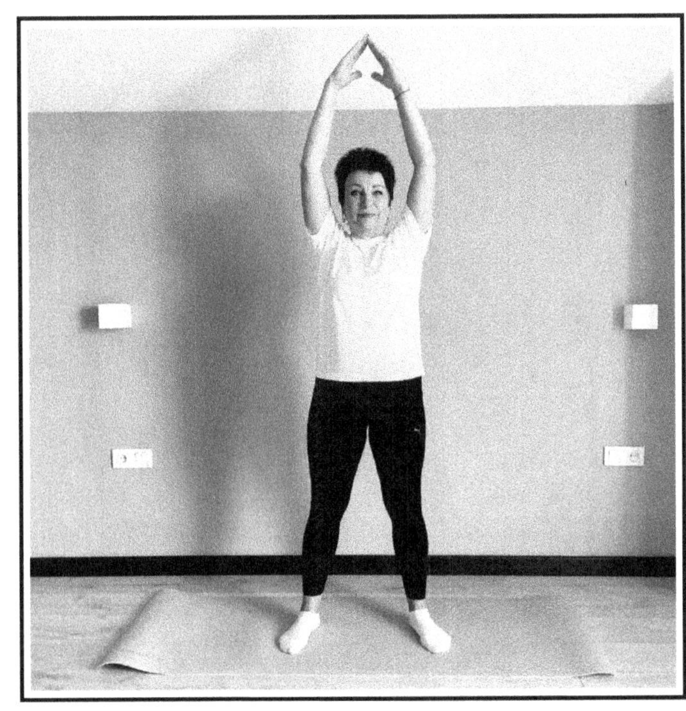 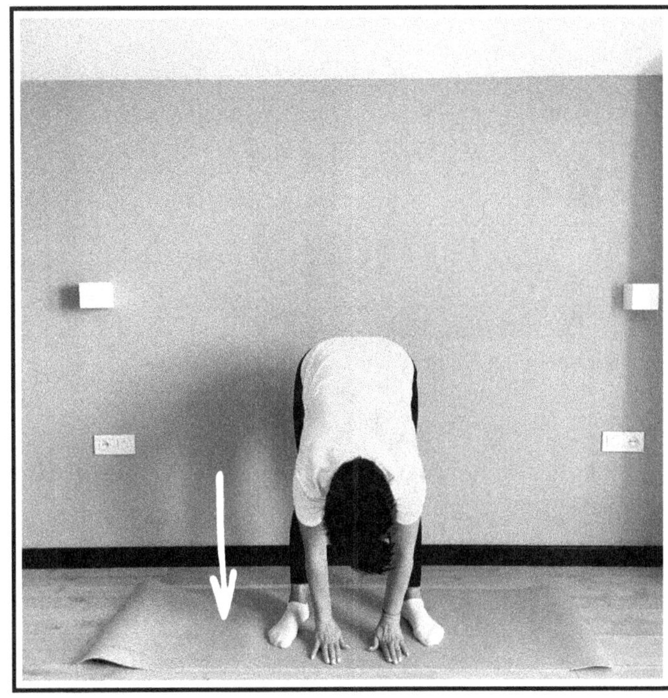

PROCEDURE:

1. Stand with your feet as wide as they can comfortably go and lift your arms straight up above your head
2. Lean forward and reach your hands toward the floor
3. Raise your torso and reach up above your head again
4. Repeat the exercise

SUGGESTED TIPS:

- Don't bend your knees; try to keep them as straight as possible and bend only at the waist
- Reach as far as comfortable, making sure the glutes are engaged as you stand up
- Don't arch your back

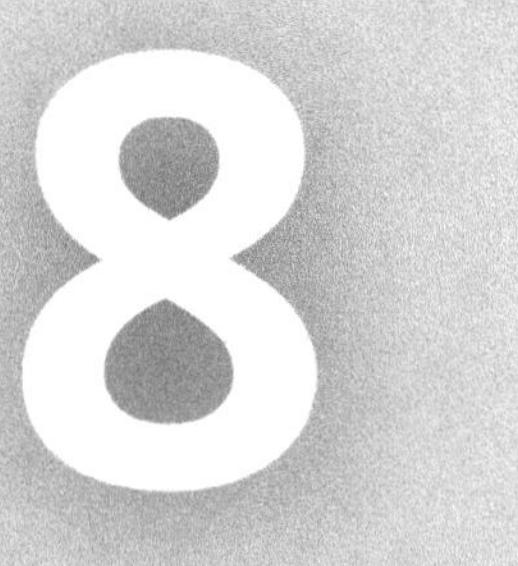

Windmill

This standing midsection exercise rotates toe touches and builds a strong link between the upper and lower body.

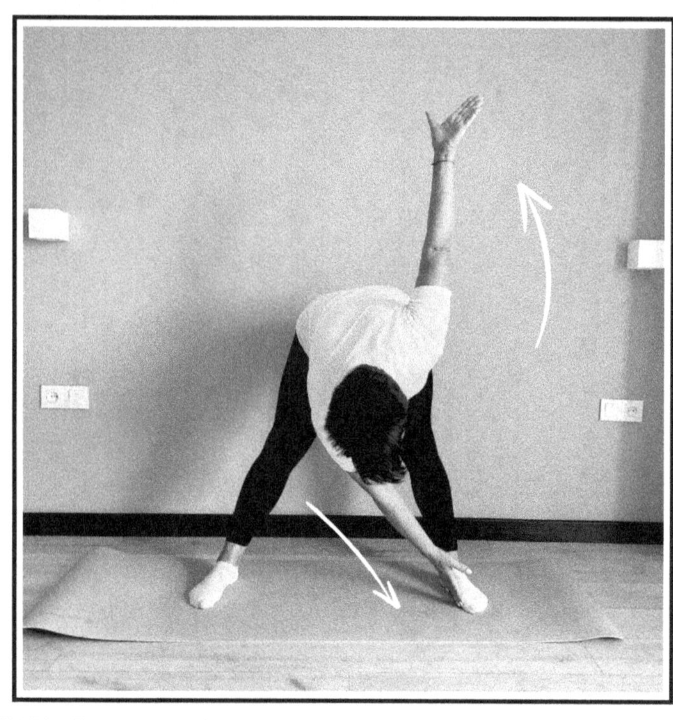 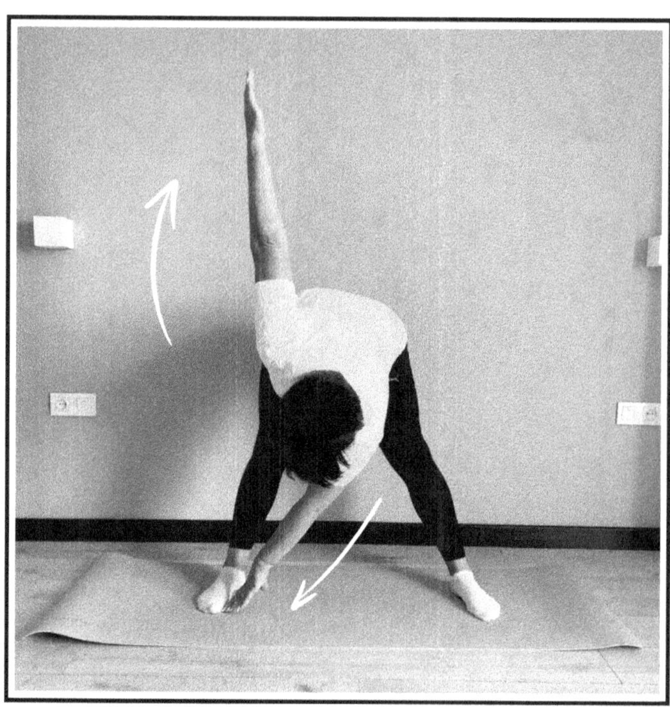

PROCEDURE:

1. Stand with your feet wider than shoulder-width and arms out to the sides parallel to the floor
2. Bend down and simultaneously rotate your upper body to the right side to touch the right toe with your left hand
3. Return to the starting position
4. Alternate between sides

SUGGESTED TIPS:

- Don't round your back
- Don't go too fast; perform slow, controlled movements to work the abdominal muscles and avoid injury
- Keep your back straight and chest up throughout the exercise

Roll Down

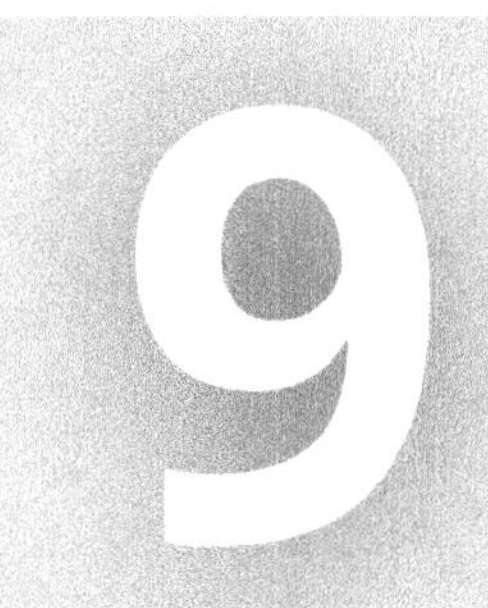

Doing crunches in a standing position helps to relax and stretch your muscles.

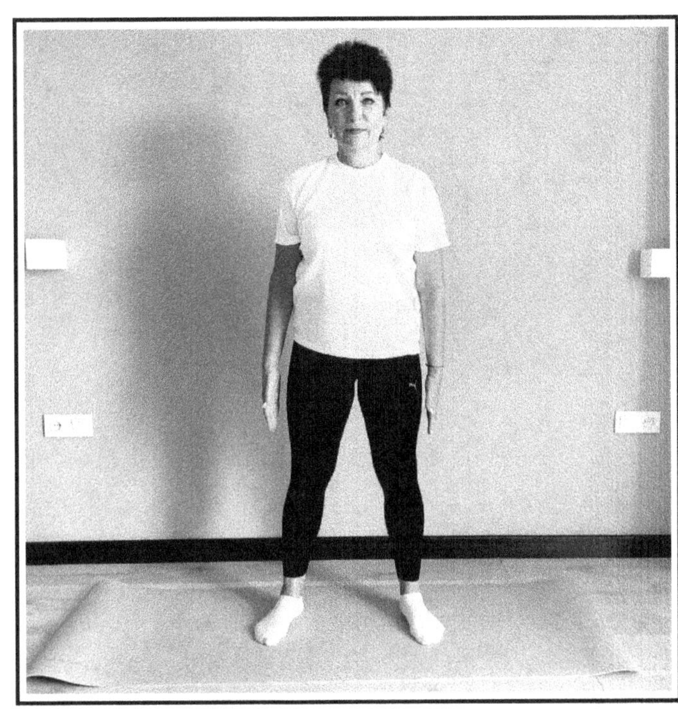

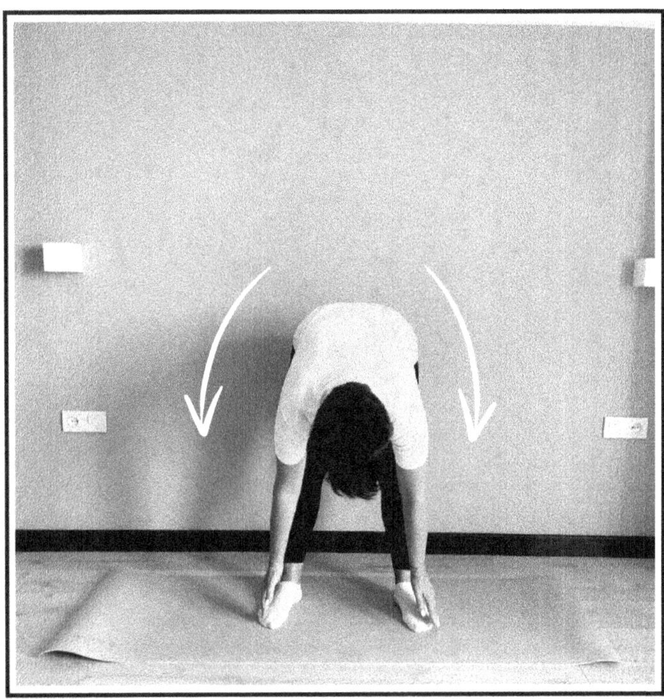

1. Stand tall with your feet hip-width apart
2. Let your arms and head slowly drop toward the floor
3. Bend your upper and lower back while your arms move downward
4. Go back up slowly
5. Repeat the movement

- Don't rush the movement
- Don't hold the breath
- Inhale at the beginning of the movement; start exhaling slowly while your arms are dropping downward

Banded Thoracic Rotations

This simple exercise simultaneously tones your arms and core.

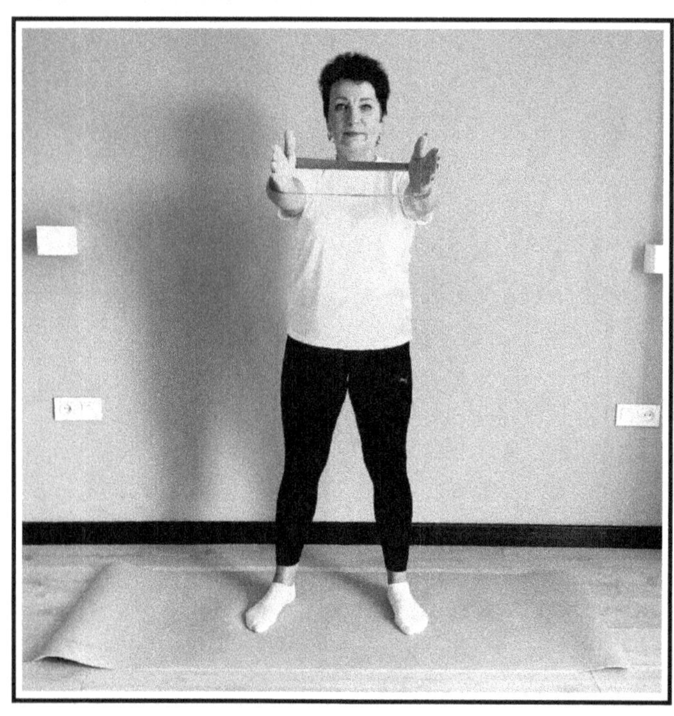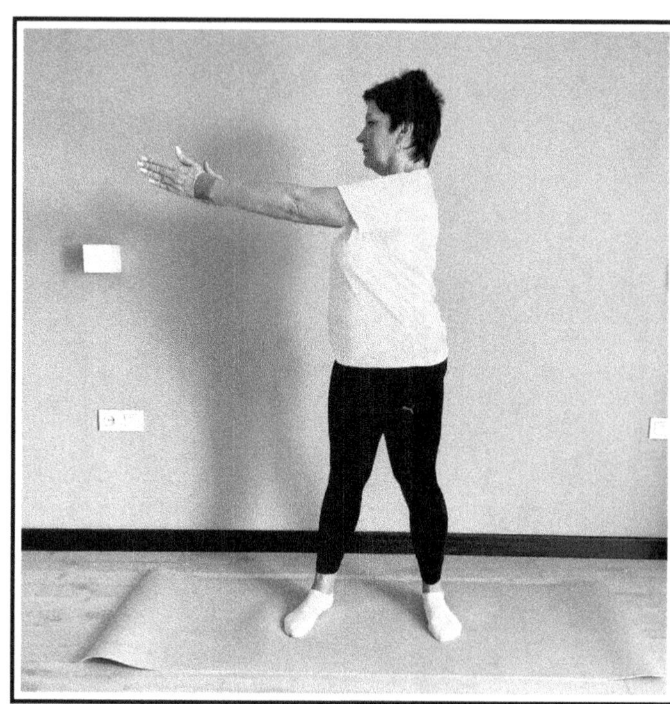

PROCEDURE:

1. Stand tall with your chest up and abs engaged
2. Put your arms out straight in front of you; place a loop band above your wrists and stretch it
3. Rotate your torso to one side and then back across to the other while keeping your hips facing forward
4. Alternate between sides

SUGGESTED TIPS:

- Don't rush; have slow, controlled movement (avoid jerking)
- Don't push yourself too hard but perform the movement in a full range of motion

Overhead Reach Side-to-Side

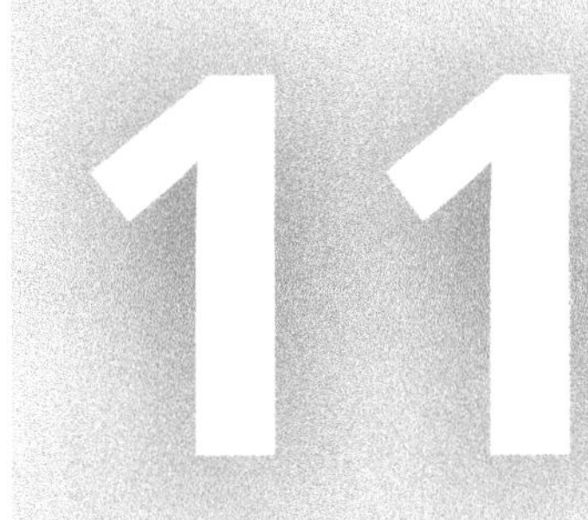

This exercise can be done anywhere. It helps stretch your core and the upper and lower back. It also relieves tension in your shoulders, back, and neck.

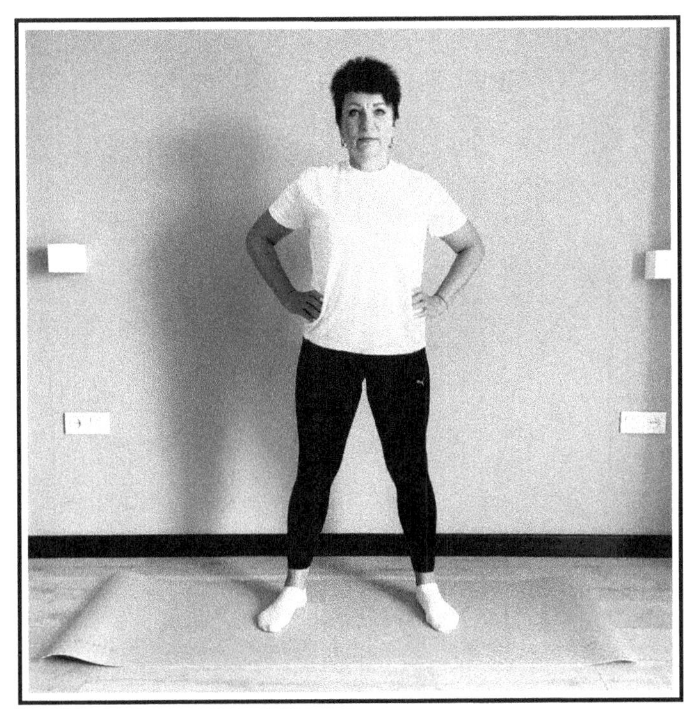
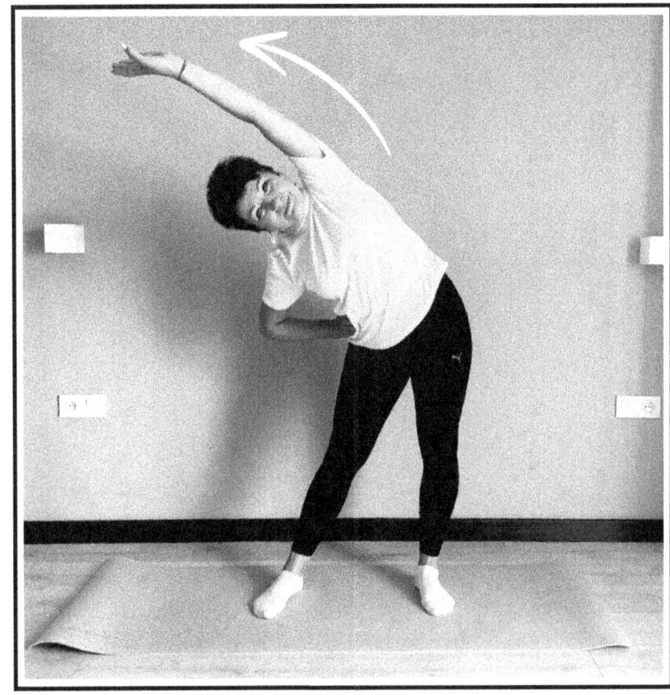

PROCEDURE:

1. Stand with feet a little wider than shoulder-width apart and both hands on hips
2. Leave one hand on the hip; reach the other arm up and over your body to feel a stretch
3. Hold for 1-2 seconds; return to the starting position with both hands on the hips
4. Alternate between sides

SUGGESTED TIPS:

- Don't lean forward or back
- Breathe deeply throughout the stretch to keep the body relaxed
- Avoid quick and jerky movements as this can cause pain and injury

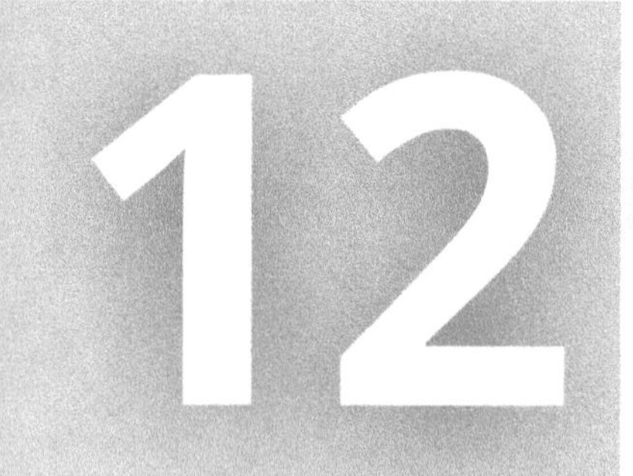

12 Chest Openers

This is a great exercise for stretching your chest and shoulder muscles.

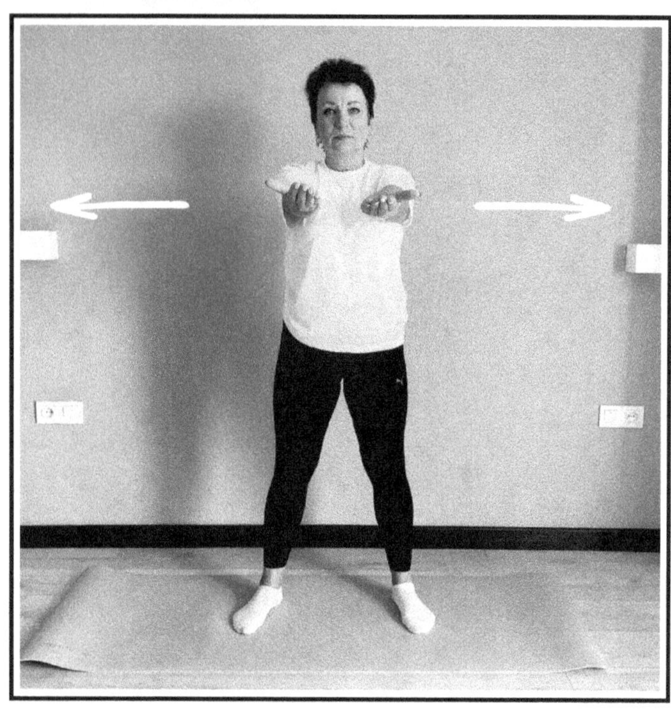

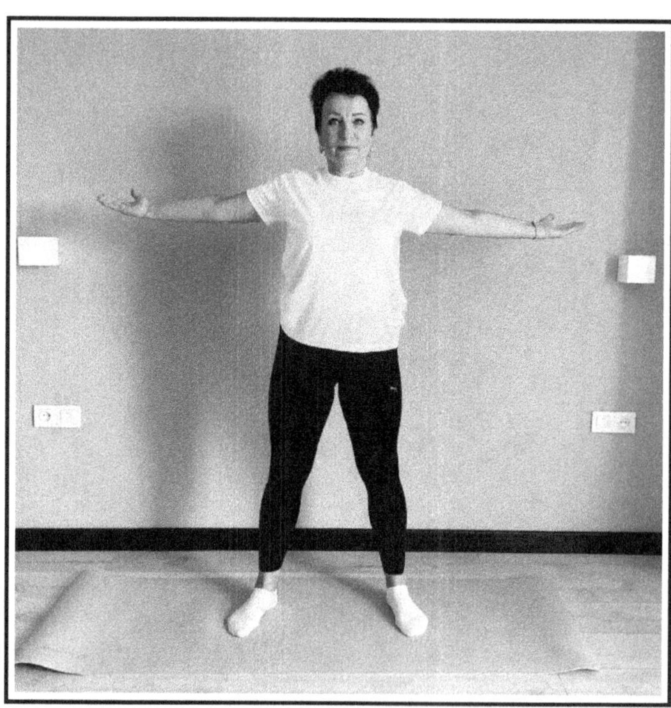

1. Stand straight with your arms in front with your palms up
2. Inhale and spread your arms back
3. Open up your chest and shoulders; squeeze the shoulder blades
4. Return to the starting position
5. Repeat the movement

- Make sure to spread the arms out and open up the chest enough
- When inhaling, move your arms out and back
- When exhaling, bring the arms together
- Squeeze the shoulder blades and feel the stretch in the chest muscles

Hurdle Steps

This excellent bodyweight exercise targets your lower body and core muscles while improving your range of motion and hip mobility.

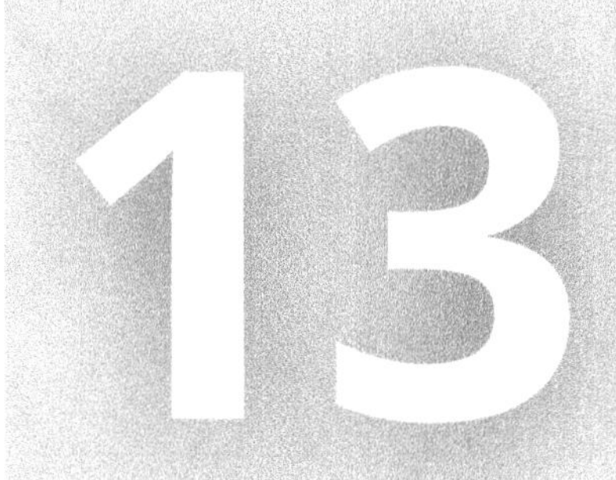

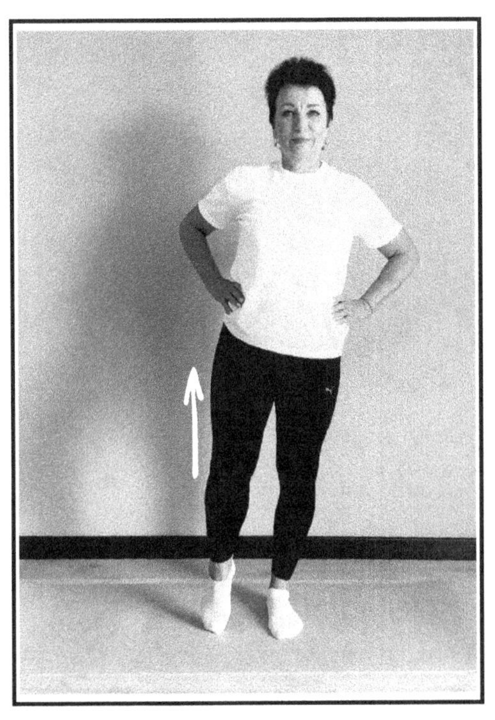
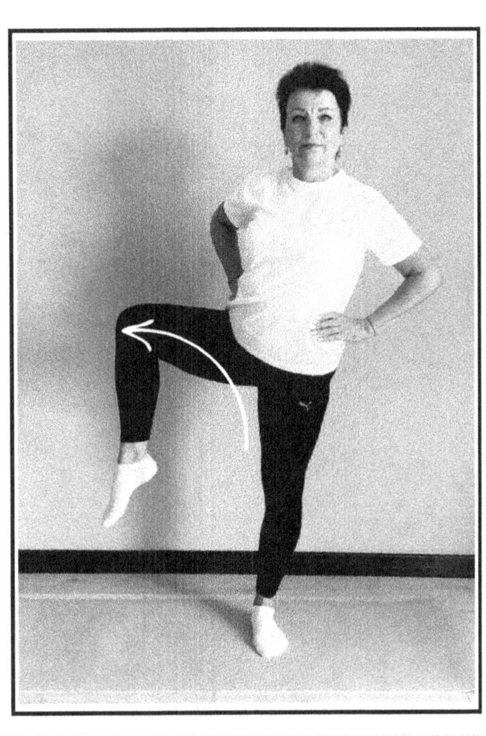
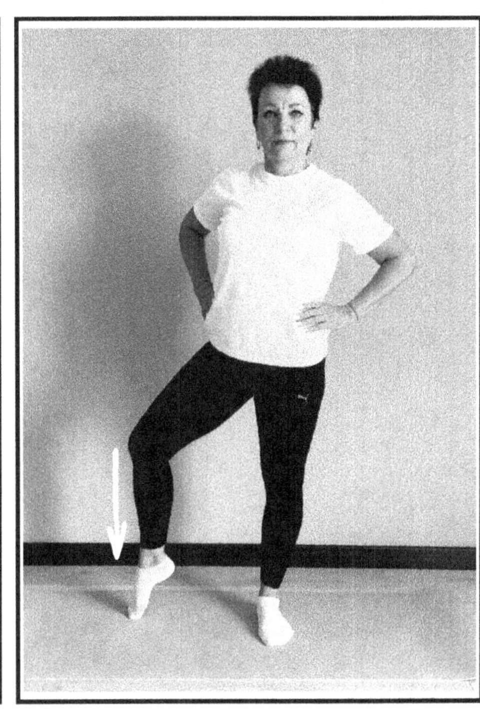

PROCEDURE:

1. Stand tall with your hands on the hips
2. Lift your left knee to waist height; flex the foot
3. Move the knee out to the side to open the hip as far as possible
4. Bring your foot to the floor; lift your knee again
5. Reverse the movement; bring your leg back to the middle and drop the foot to the floor
6. Alternate between legs

SUGGESTED TIPS:

- Don't go too fast
- Don't relax the core; don't round the back
- Don't twist the body when lifting and opening the leg; keep the body pointed forward, engage the core, and straighten the back

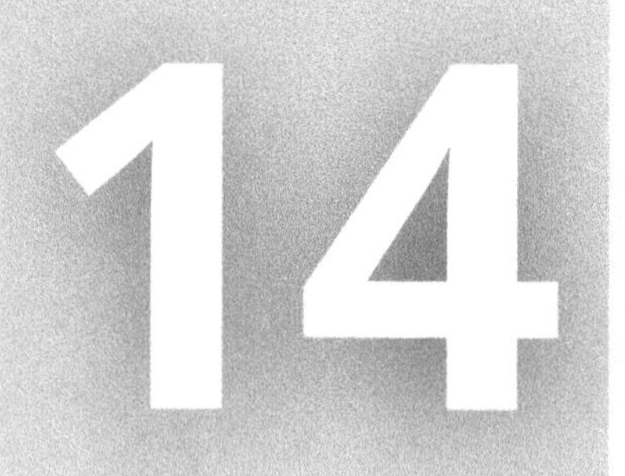

Side Leg Raise with Heel Touch
(Right, Left)

This is one of the most effective exercises for strength building in your glutes, hips, abs, and thighs.

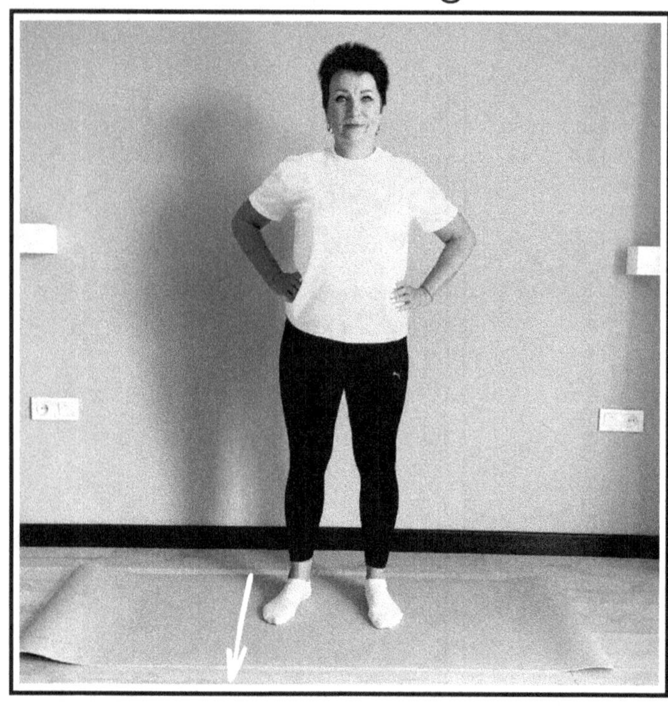

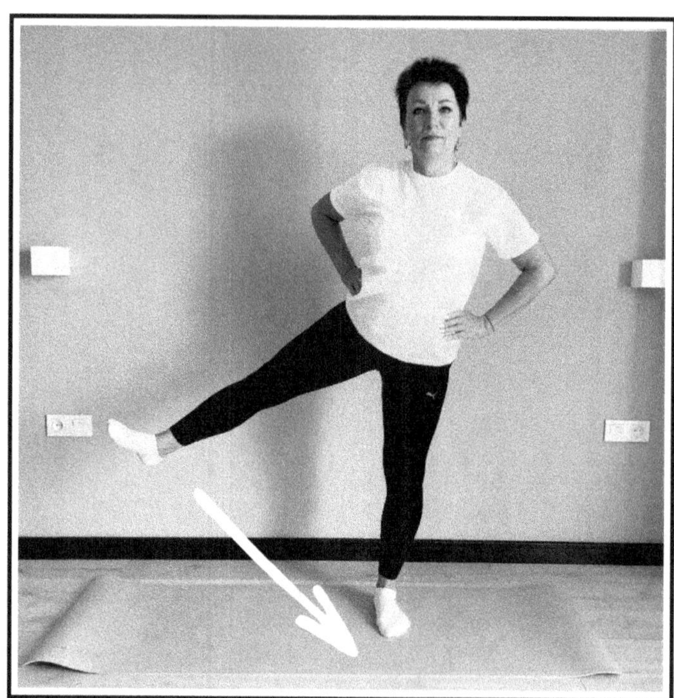

1. Stand with your hands on the hips
2. Step forward with the right leg on your heel; keep both legs leg straight
3. Lift the right leg out toward the side; swing it back down
4. Repeat the movement
5. Perform the exercise using the left leg

- Don't round the lower back
- Don't relax the core
- Keep the back straight

Standing Rotations

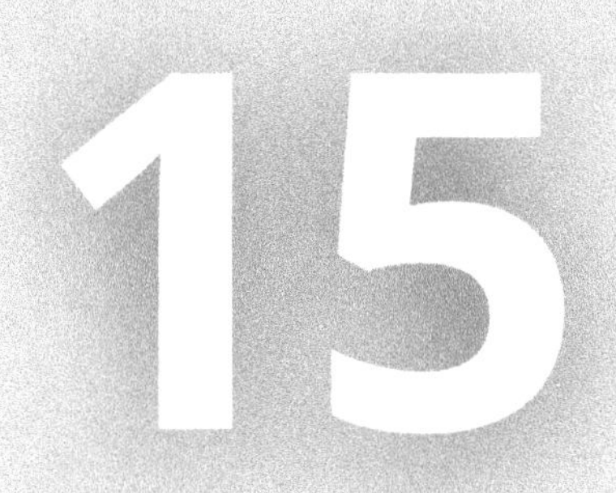

This simple exercise will simultaneously tone your arms and core.

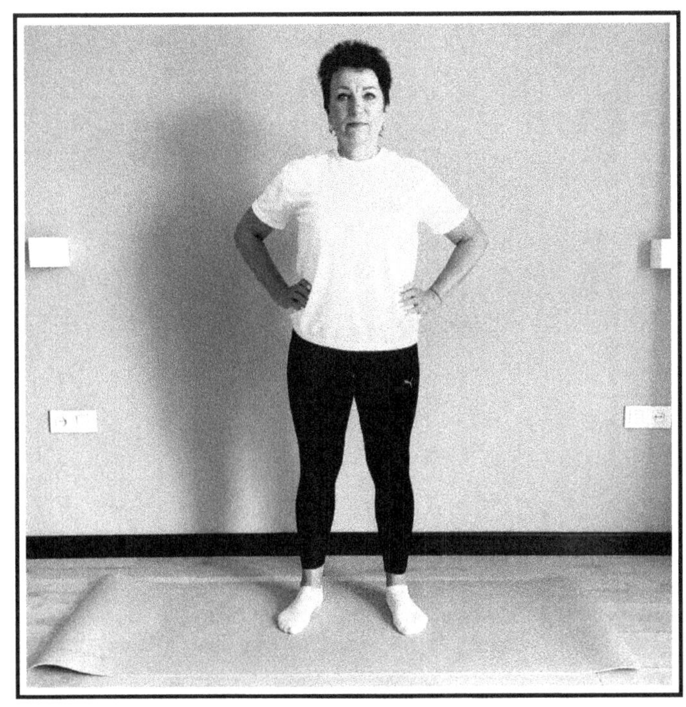
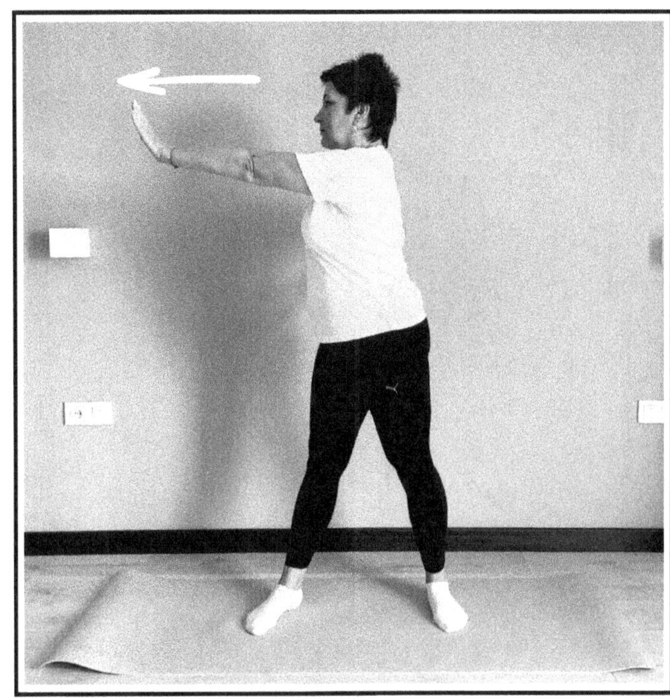

PROCEDURE:

1. Stand with your hands on the hips
2. Reach one arm across your body twisting at the waist
3. Repeat with the opposite arm reaching toward the opposite side
4. Alternate between sides

SUGGESTED TIPS:

- Your arms should not be doing all the work; twist as far as your hips will comfortably go
- Maintain a good pace; don't go too fast that your form suffers

Robot Arms

Robot Arms is a great exercise to work the rotator cuff muscles and shoulder mobility (internal and external).

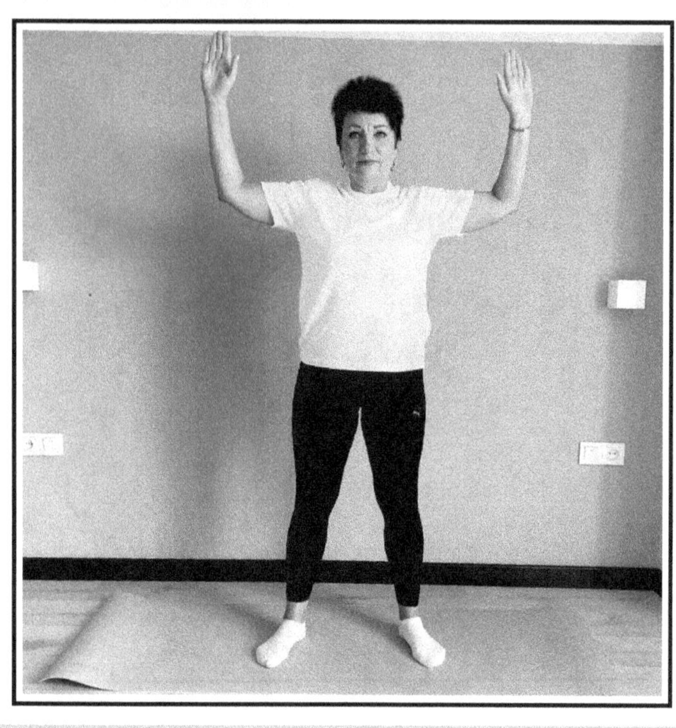
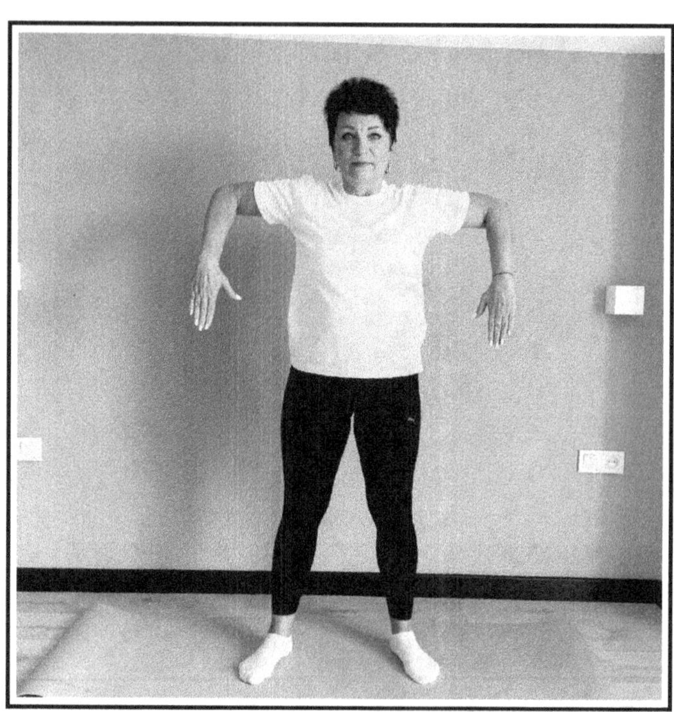

PROCEDURE:

1. Stand up tall
2. Place the elbows at a 90-degree angle with your fingers pointing up
3. Rotate the arms down slowly; fingers will be pointing down
4. Go back up; repeat the exercise

SUGGESTED TIPS:

- Go slowly
- Keep the elbows at a 90-degree all the time

Upper Body Exercises

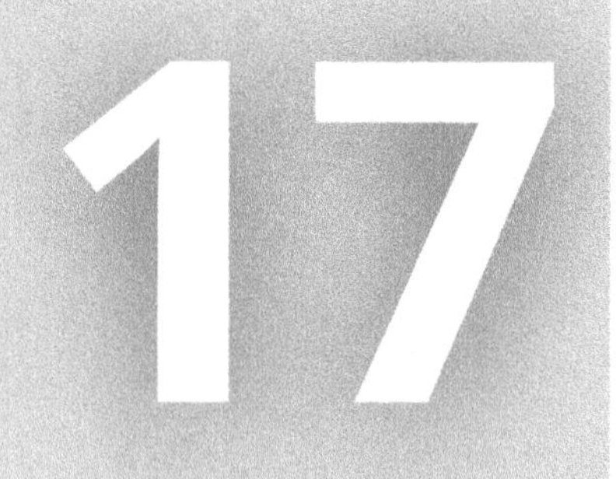

Arm Raises with a Band

This exercise is fantastic for improving shoulder mobility, especially after a long sitting session.

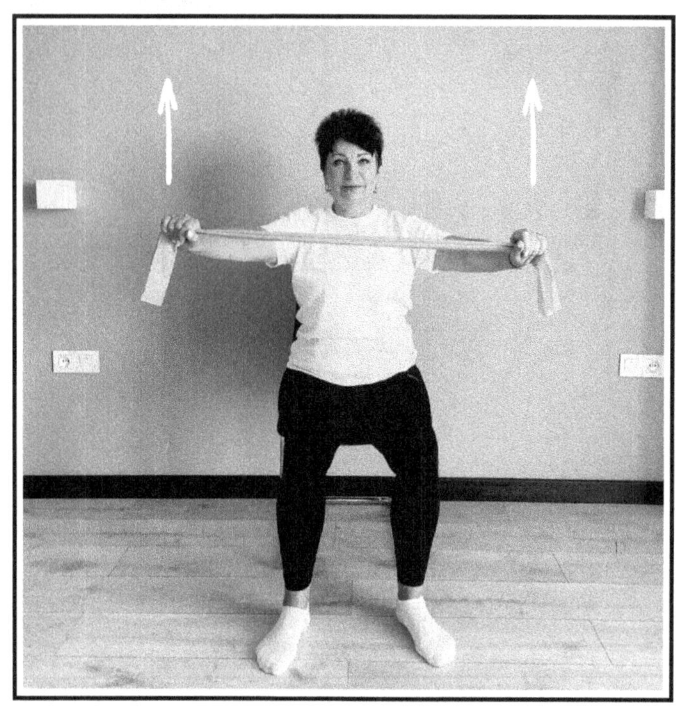

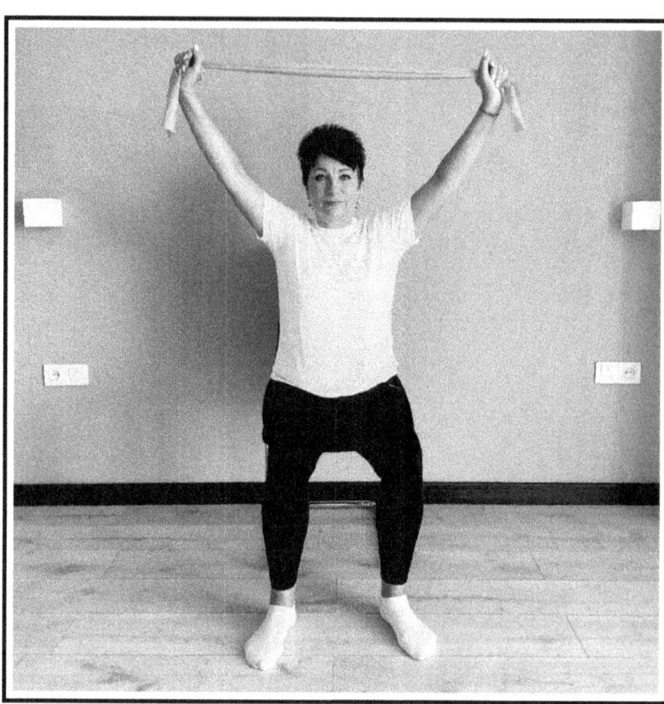

PROCEDURE:

1. Sit on a chair with your hands shoulder-width apart
2. Stretch the band in front of you
3. Lift your arms over your head
4. Bring the arms back
5. Repeat the movement

SUGGESTED TIPS:

- Don't move too fast
- Don't bend the arms
- At the beginning of the movement, inhale; as you bring your arms over your head, slowly exhale

PAGE 36

Chair Diagonal Stretch

This exercise is perfect for activating your back muscles and stretching your biceps. It also stretches the pectoral and shoulder muscles.

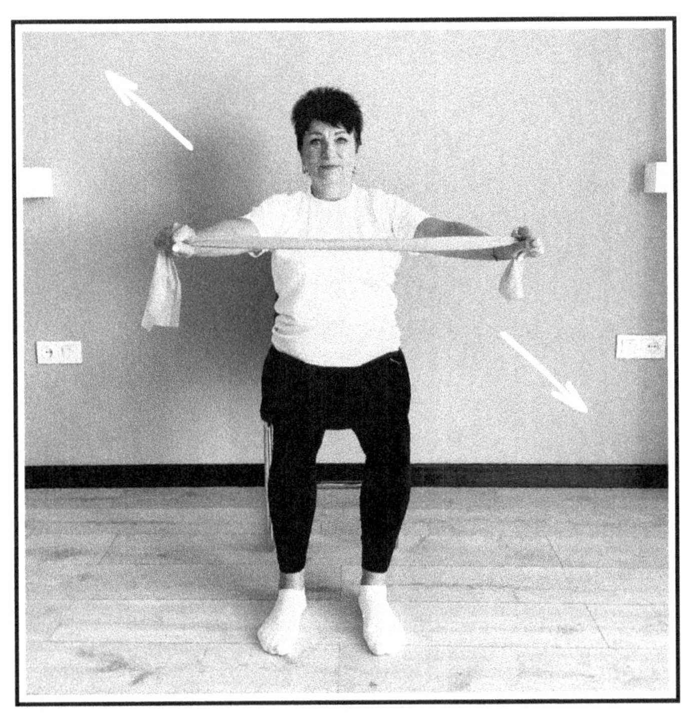
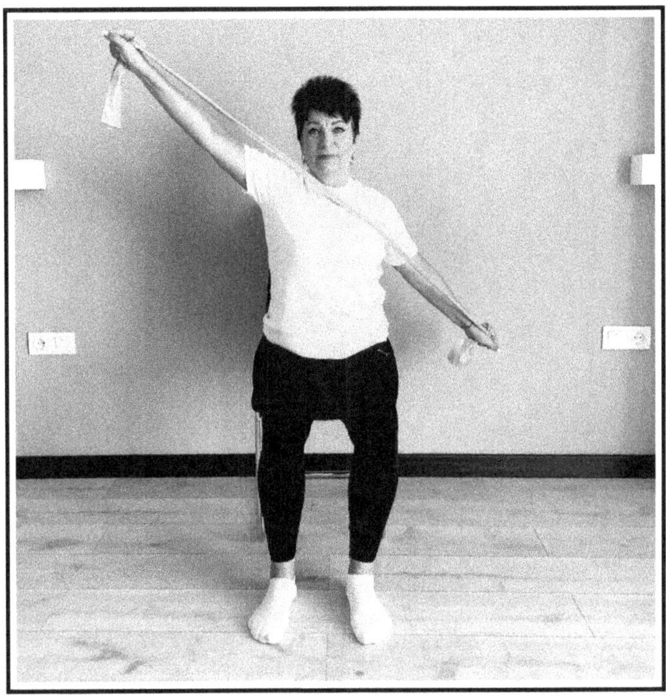

PROCEDURE:

1. Sit tall on a chair
2. Hold the resistance band in your hands while extending your arms forward
3. Then stretch the band diagonally
4. Go back up to the previous position
5. Alternate between sides

SUGGESTED TIPS:

- Don't hold the breath
- Don't rush the movement
- At the beginning of the movesment, inhale; as you stretch the band, exhale

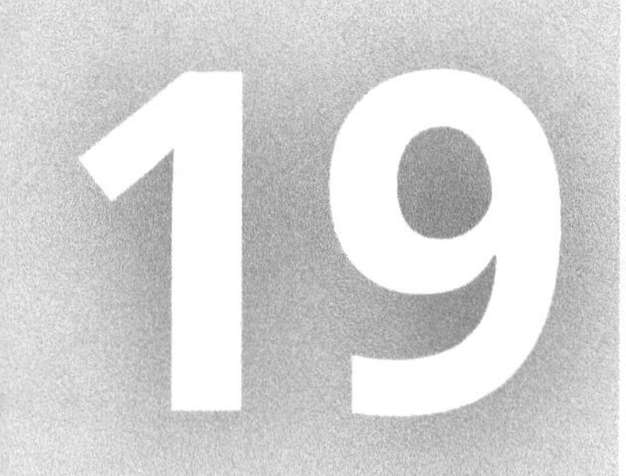

19 Banded Side Bends

The exercise helps to target your side abs from different angles.

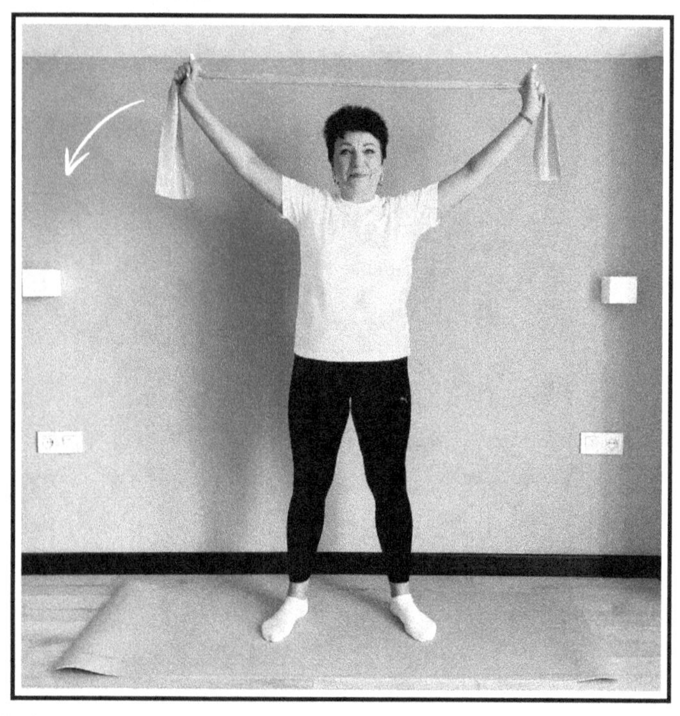

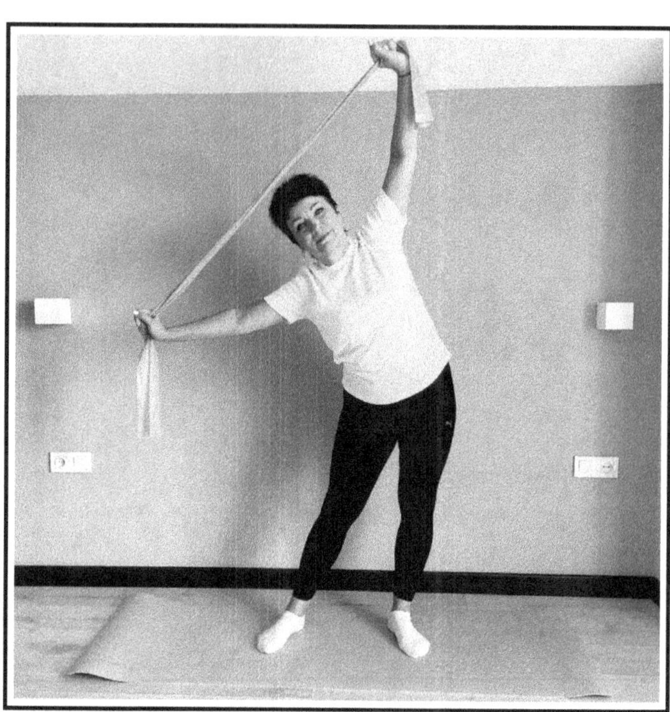

PROCEDURE:

1. Stand up straight with your feet hip-width apart
2. Fold the band and grasp both ends
3. Extend your arms overhead and stretch the band as much as possible
4. Bend your body against the resistance of the band to one side while keeping your arms extended and the band stretched
5. Before bending to the other side, slowly come back to the middle
6. Alternate between sides

SUGGESTED TIPS:

- Don't bend forward or backward
- Keep your core engaged throughout the exercise

Banded Pull Downs

This exercise helps you build a stronger back and improves your posture by maximizing the contraction of the upper muscles.

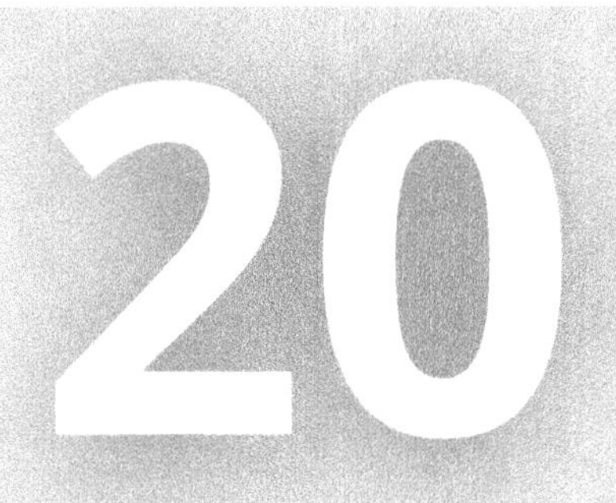

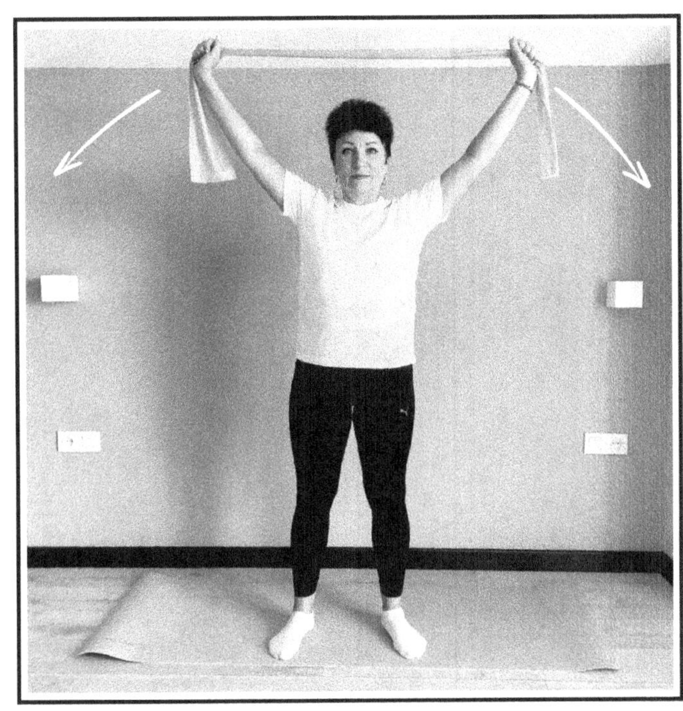 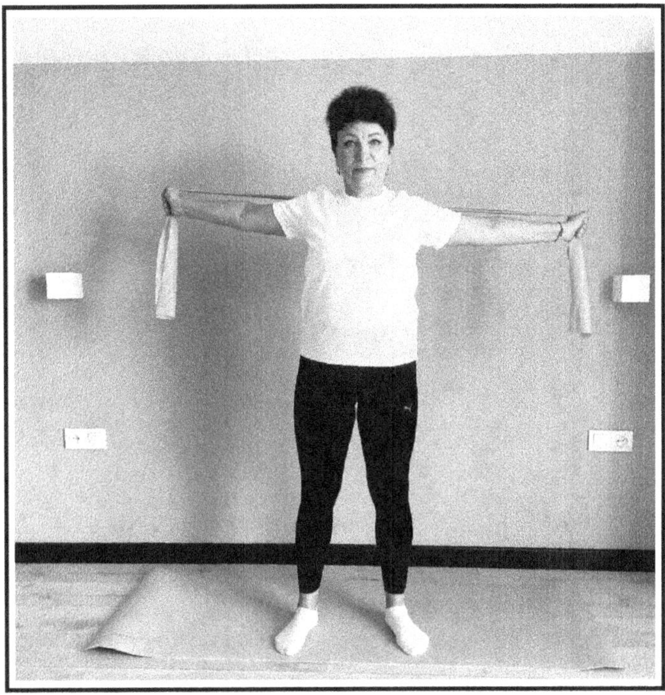

PROCEDURE:

1. Stand up straight, feet hip-width apart
2. Grasp both ends of the band
3. Activate your core while bringing your arms overhead until the band is fully stretched
4. Stretch the band behind your head until it reaches your neck
5. Go back up
6. Repeat the movement

SUGGESTED TIPS:

- Don't arch your back
- Keep the band fully stretched throughout the exercise
- When pulling the band, use your upper and middle back

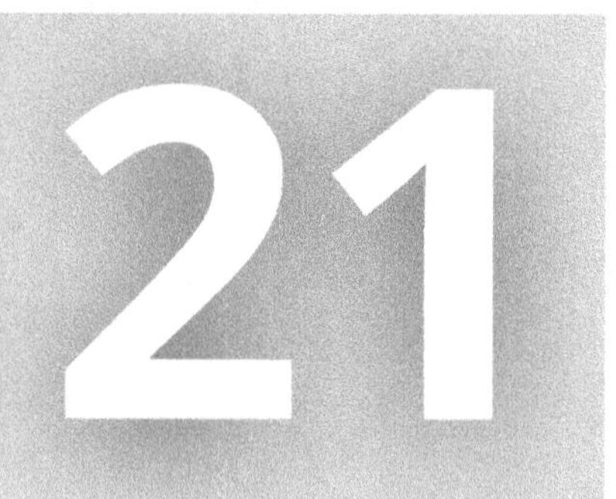

21 Arms Overhead Swing with a Band

This exercise is great for improving shoulder mobility and health. Gymnasts often use this exercise as part of their warm-up routine.

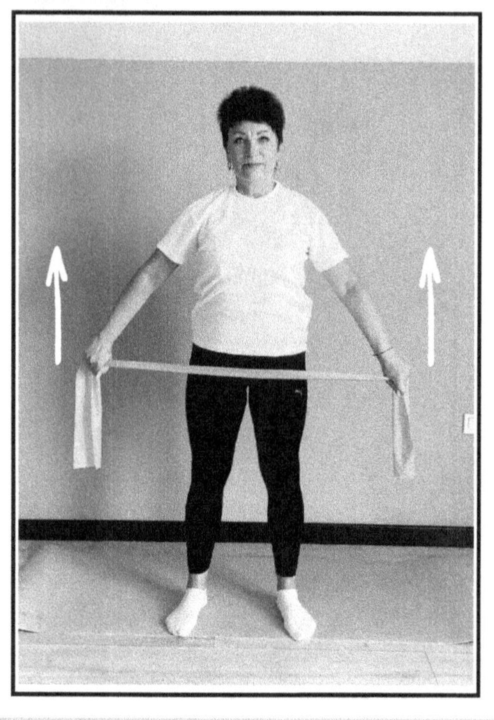 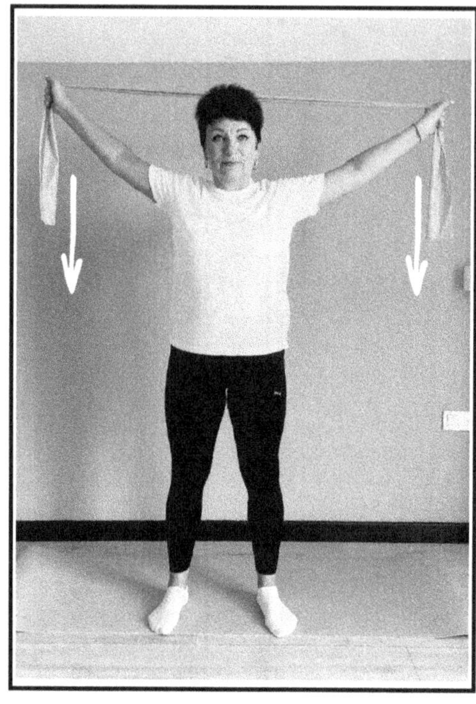 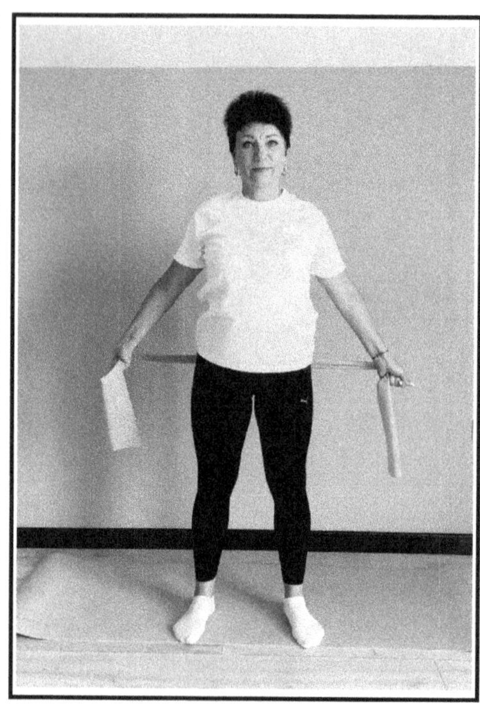

PROCEDURE:

1. Start the movement from a standing position
2. Keep your arms extended and a little wider than shoulder-width apart; slightly stretch the band
3. Perform a backward arm circle as you keep your arms extended
4. Let the band touch the glutes, and then go back up until it touches your thighs; repeat the movement

SUGGESTED TIPS:

- Don't bend the arms
- Don't arch your lower back
- Perform the move in the full range of motion
- Take a deep breath through the nose and slowly exhale as you are going down

PAGE 40

Chest Mobility with a Band

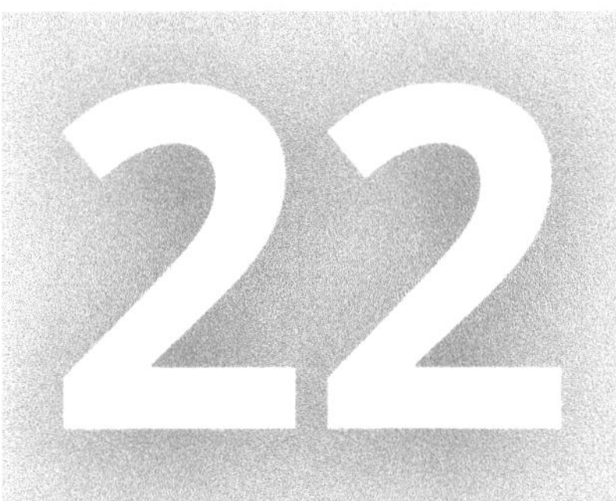

This exercise stretches your chest, activates your back muscles, and works your thoracal spine mobility.

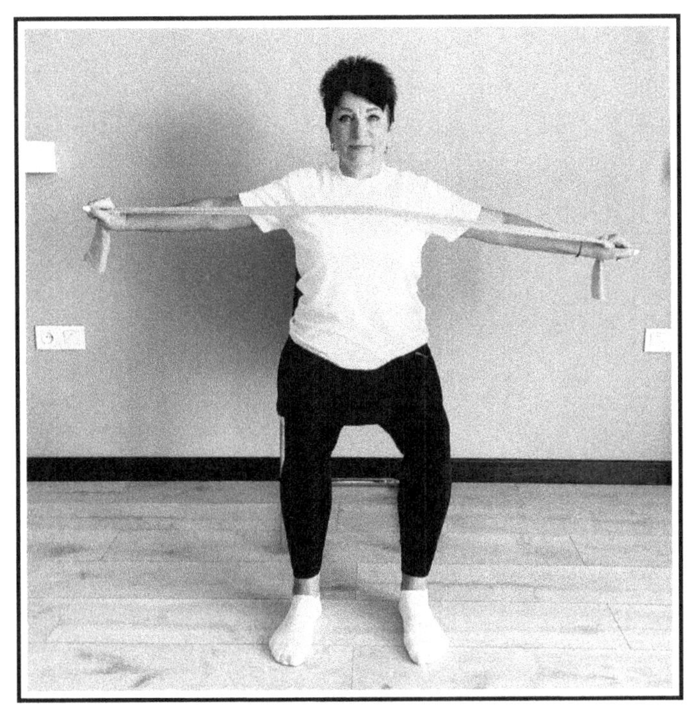 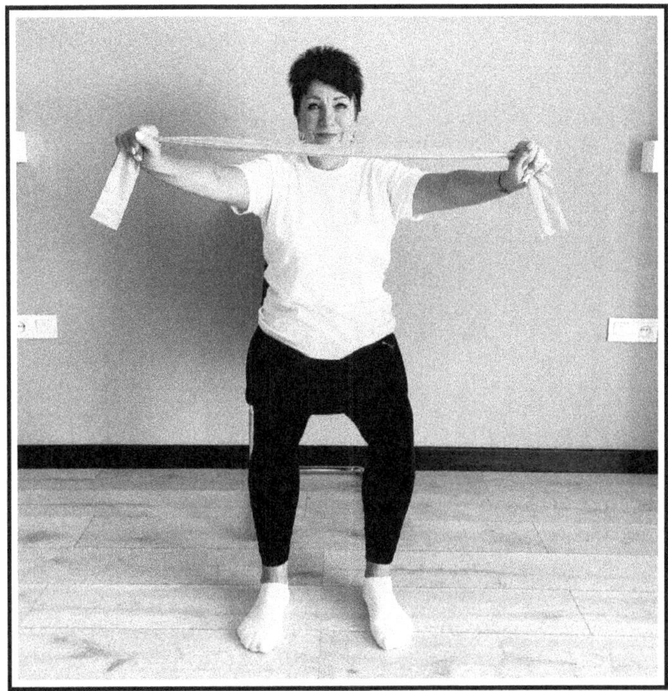

1. Sit tall on a chair
2. Grab the band and pull it across your chest
3. At the same time, stick your chest out and slightly arch your back
4. Then bend forward and round your spine
5. Repeat the movement

- Don't go too fast
- Don't hold the breath
- At the beginning of the movement, inhale; as you extend your chest out, exhale (make sure you follow the movement with your head)

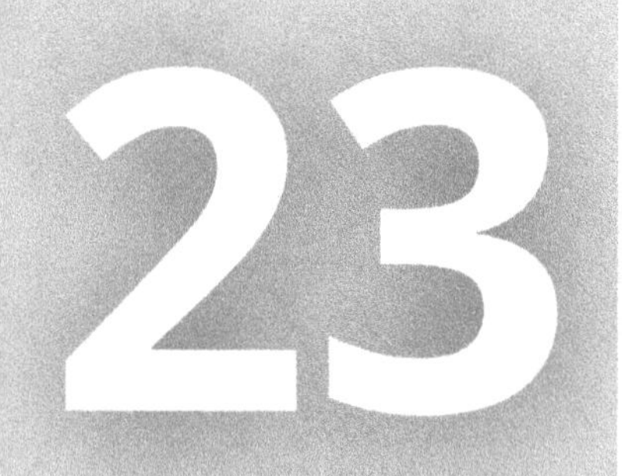

23 Overhead Arm Raise

This exercise works on your shoulder and pectoral muscles.

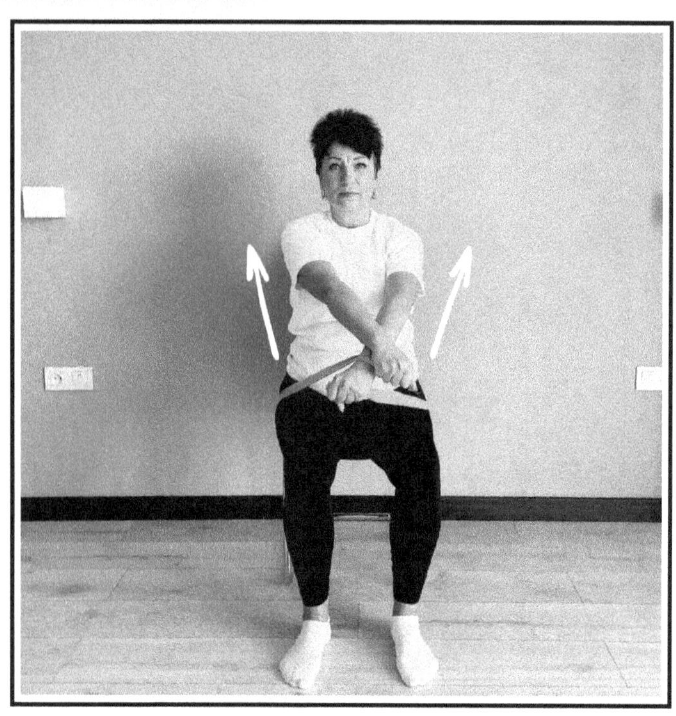

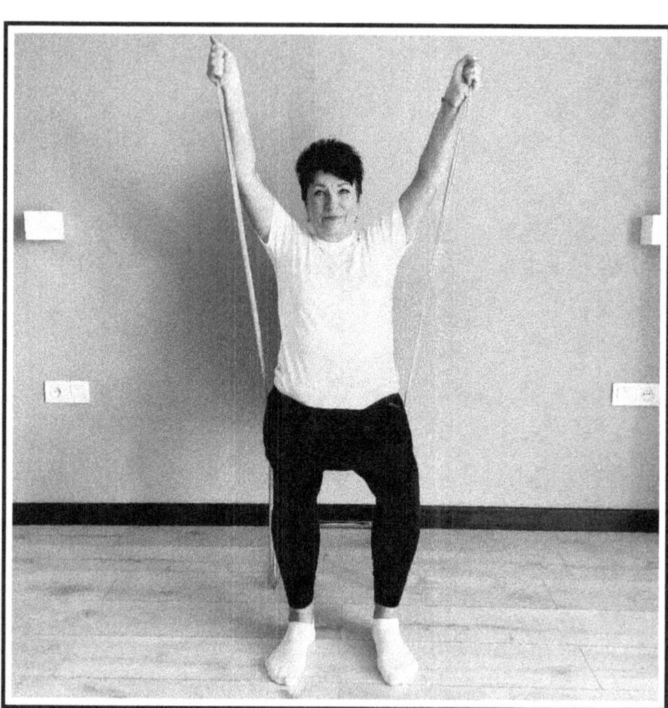

1. Sit tall on a chair and the resistance band
2. Hold the ends of the band in your hands
3. Then lift both of your arms up and above your head
4. Go down slowly and cross your arms
5. Repeat the movement

- Don't bend the arms
- Don't rush the movement
- Before you start lifting your arms, inhale; as you slowly lift, exhale

Chair-Banded Row

Chair-banded rows are phenomenal for working on your back muscles. This exercise is beneficial for improving your posture after a long day of sitting.

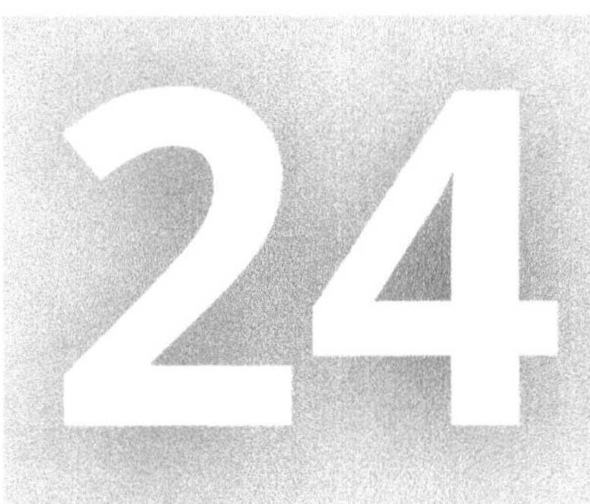

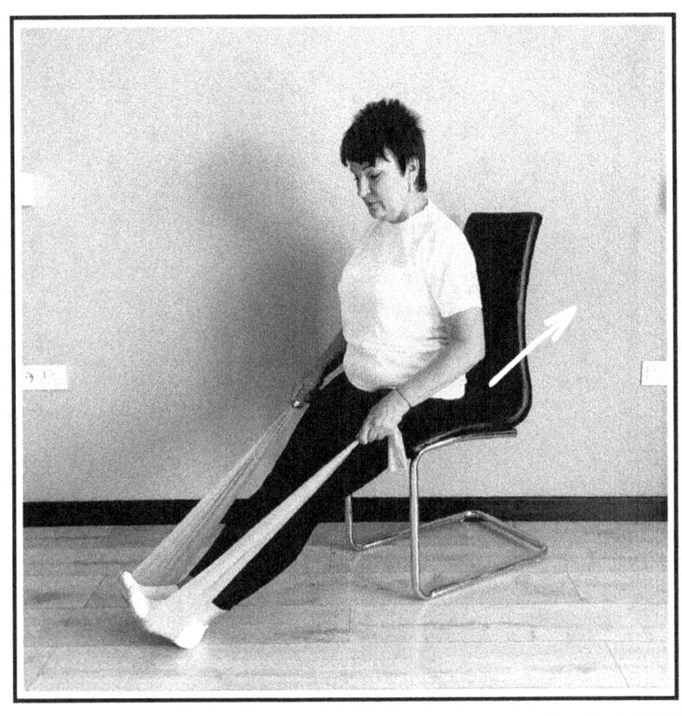

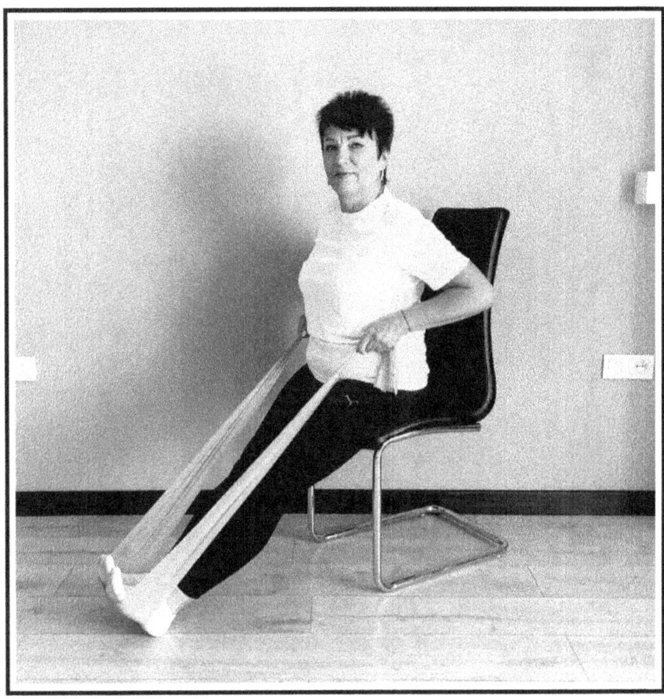

PROCEDURE:

1. Sit with your back straight on a chair
2. Put your feet together and loop the resistance band under your toes
3. Then stretch the band and squeeze the back muscles
4. Sit back up and release the resistance
5. Repeat the movement

SUGGESTED TIPS:

- Don't stretch the band too fast
- Don't arch the lower back
- Don't hold the breath
- At the beginning of the movement, inhale; as you are pulling the band, exhale
- To increase the intensity of this exercise, use a stronger band

Thoracic Rotations with Knee Raises

This is a great warm-up exercise. It can be incorporated into your pre-run routine.

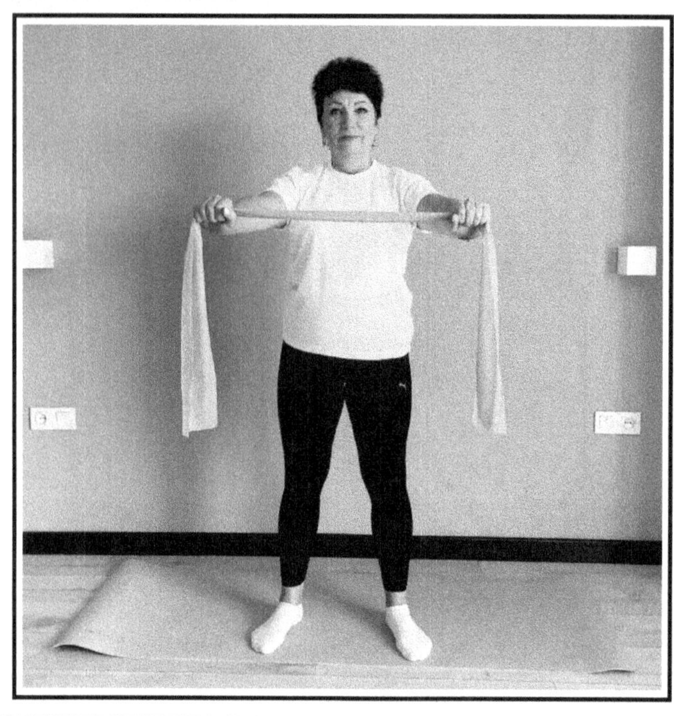 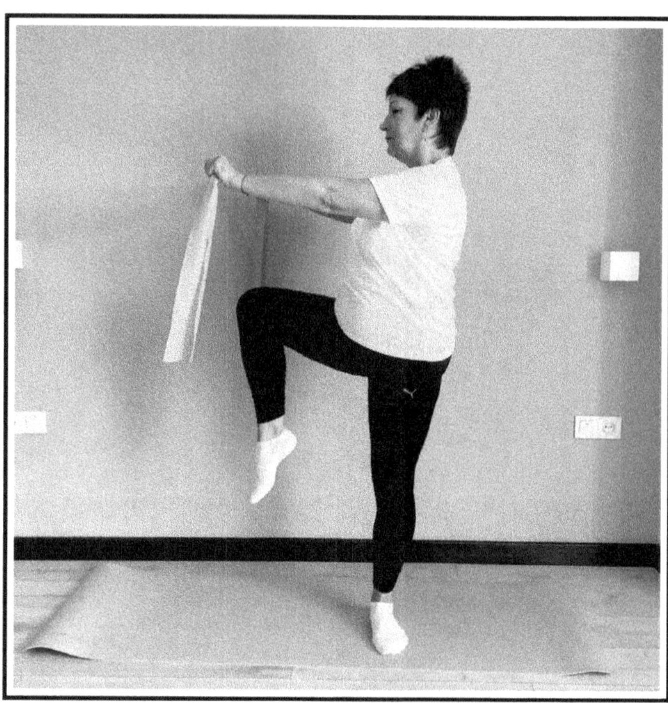

PROCEDURE:

1. Stand tall with feet shoulder-width apart; place a band above your wrists, keeping it taut
2. Extend your arms to the front of you while lifting your right knee and twisting your torso to the right side
3. Bring your right foot back and return to a standing position
4. Repeat the movement twisting your torso to the left side
5. Alternate between sides

SUGGESTED TIPS:

- Don't go too fast; keep the form
- Don't forget to breathe deeply throughout the exercise
- Go at your own pace; start slow and then increase the intensity and move faster

Banded Romanian Deadlift

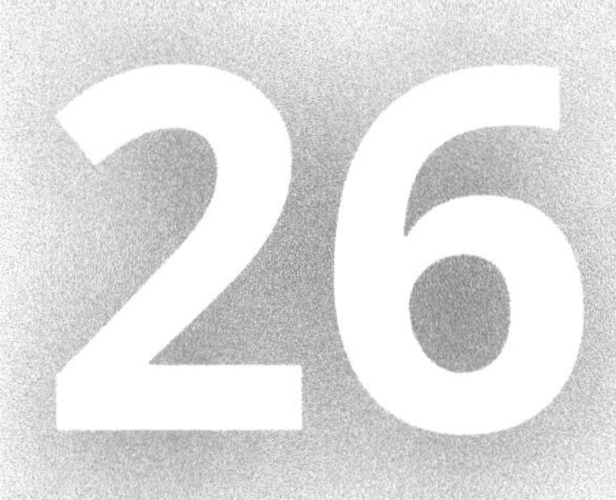

The exercise is ideal for specifically targeting the lower rhomboids to help achieve a toned upper back.

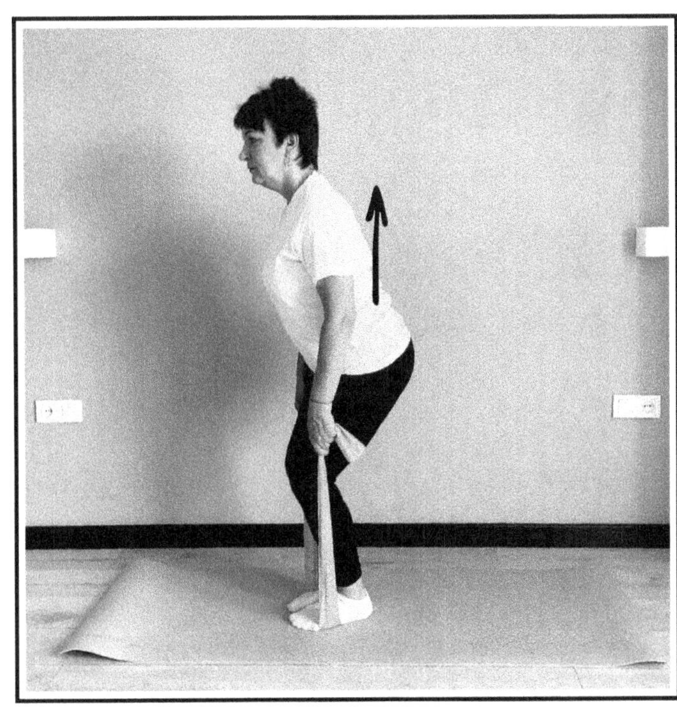 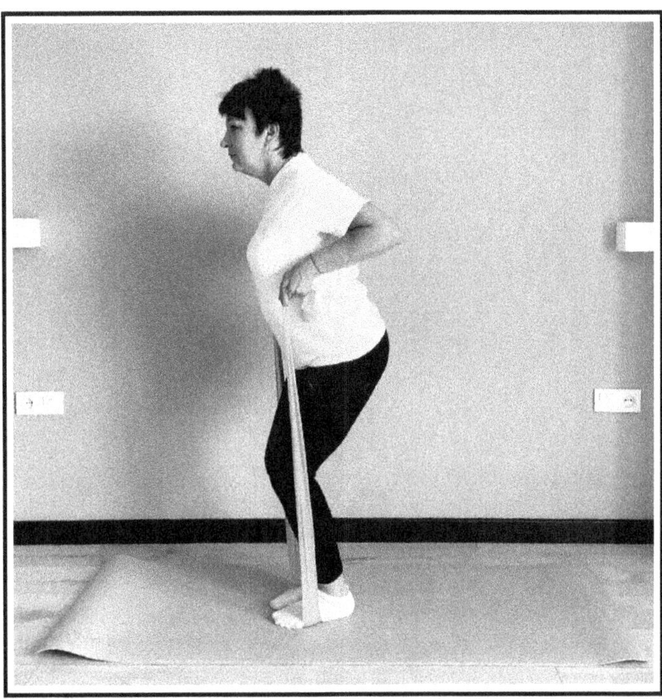

PROCEDURE:

1. With both feet, step on the band; grasp both ends
2. Keep your feet hip-width apart
3. Bend your upper body forward as you keep your core activated and back straight; slightly bend your knees
4. Slowly return to the starting position
5. Repeat the movement

SUGGESTED TIPS:

- Don't arch or round your back
- Don't relax your core
- Change to a heavier band if you can do more than 10-15 reps

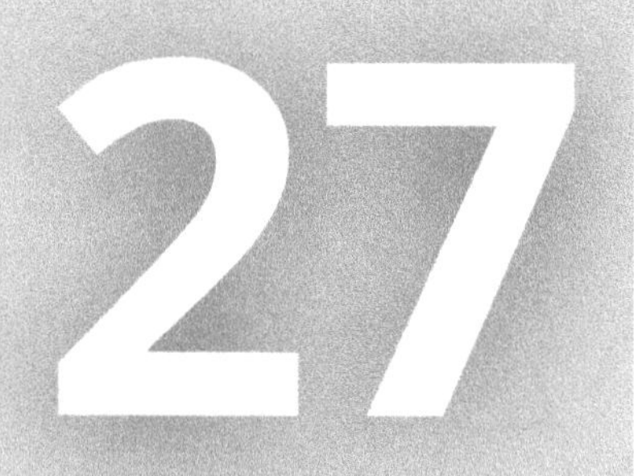

Chair-Banded Row
(Right, Left)

This exercise works your back muscles and is good for improving your posture.

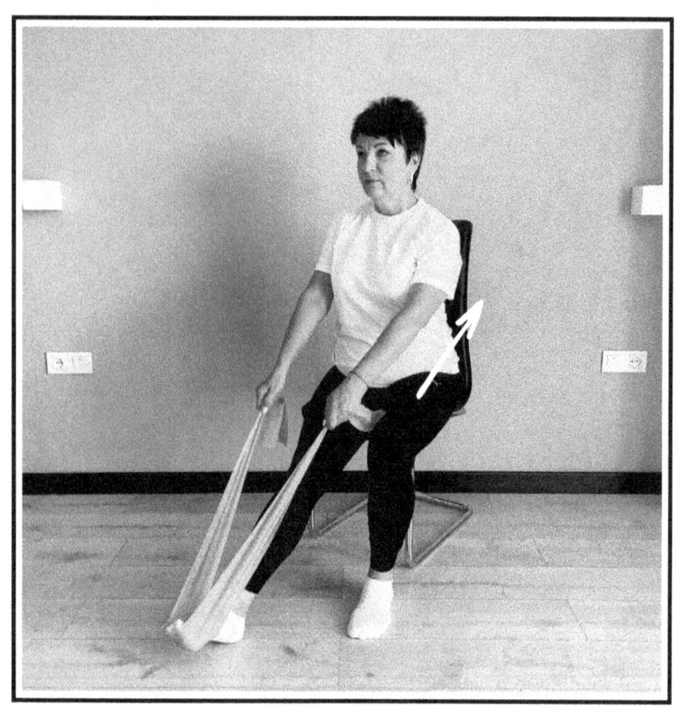
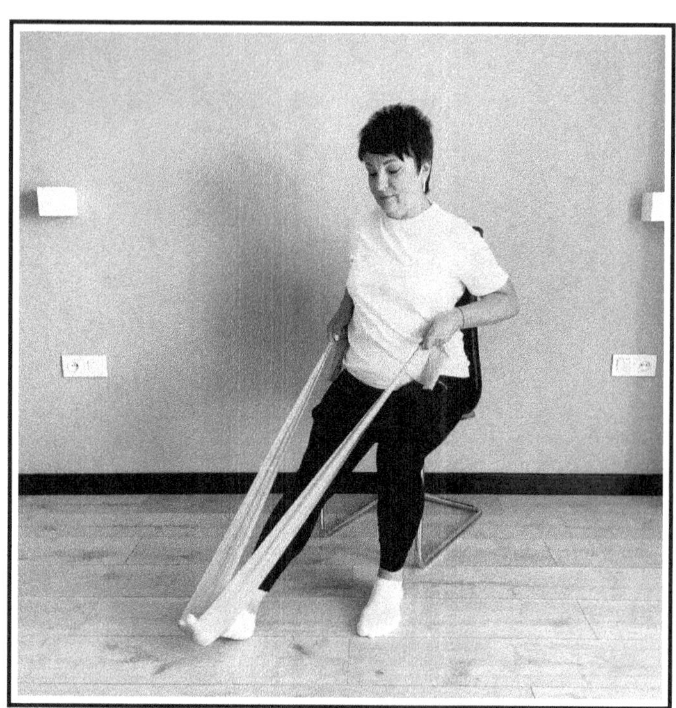

PROCEDURE:

1. Sit with your back straight on a chair
2. Extend your right foot forward and loop the resistance band under your toes
3. Then stretch the band and squeeze the back muscles
4. Sit back up and release the resistance
5. Repeat the movement
6. Perform the exercise using the other foot

SUGGESTED TIPS:

- Don't stretch the band too fast
- Don't arch the lower back
- Don't hold the breath
- At the beginning of the movement, inhale; as you are pulling the band, exhale

Banded Waiter

This exercise challenges your external shoulder function and strengthens your rotator cuff muscles.

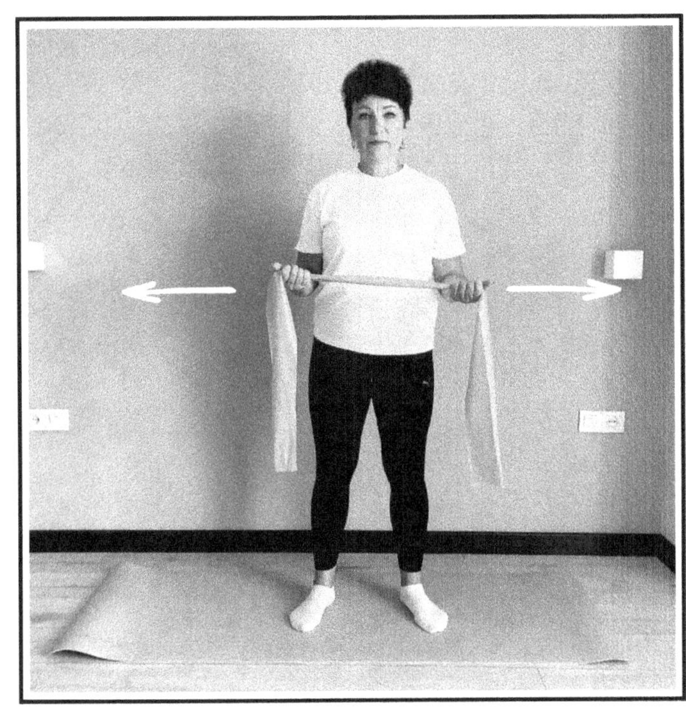

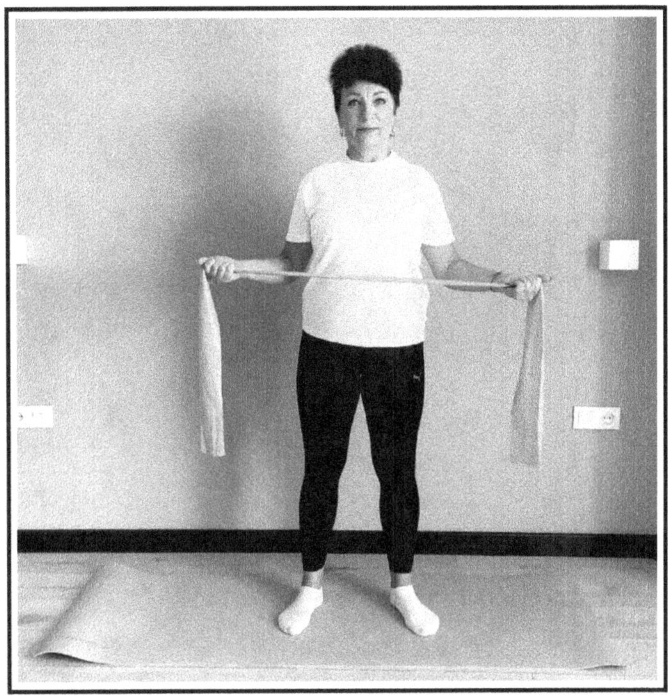

PROCEDURE:

1. Stand tall by holding the band in your hands
2. Bend your elbows at 90 degrees; keep them close to your body
3. Then stretch the band
4. Go back to the starting position
5. Repeat the movement

SUGGESTED TIPS:

- Keep the elbows bent at 90 degrees
- Don't do the exercise too fast
- Each repetition should be about 2 seconds

29 Banded Tricep Extension
(Right, Left)

This is a fantastic exercise for strengthening and stretching your triceps. It also challenges your internal shoulder rotation.

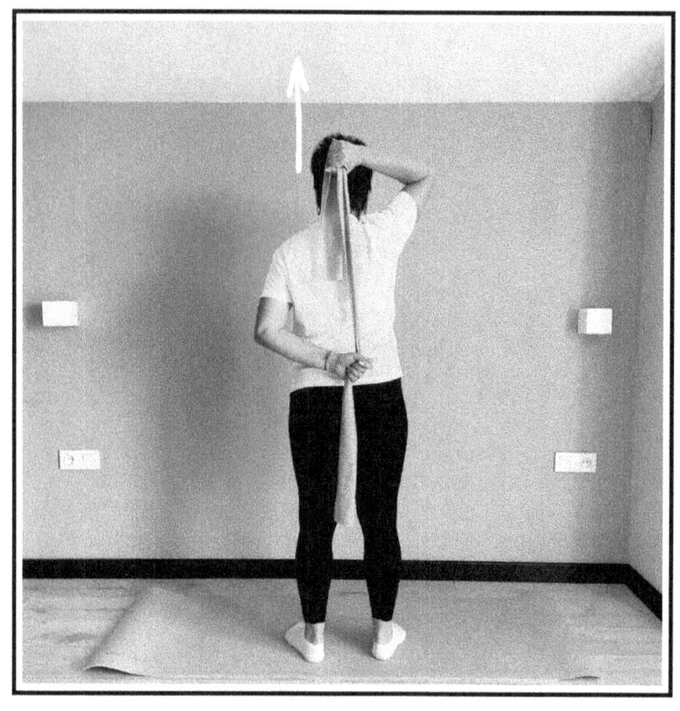

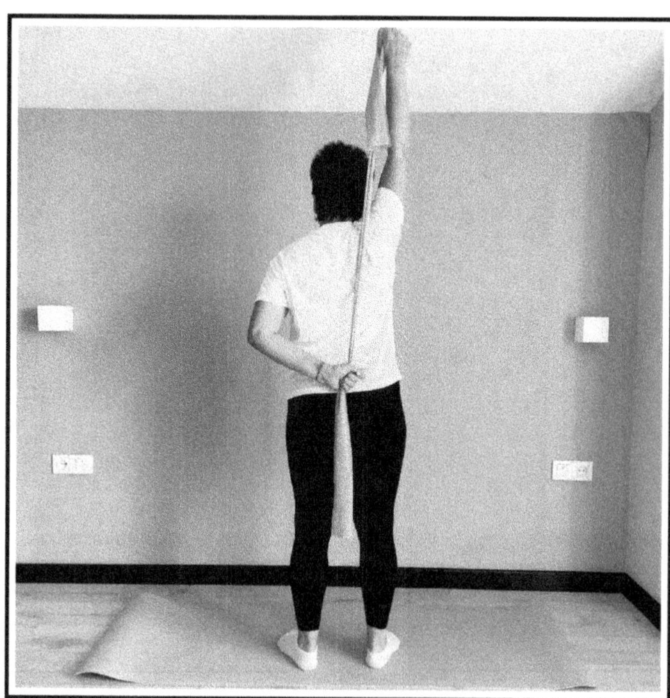

1. Stand tall and hold the band behind your back
2. Grab the bottom of the band with your left hand and the top of the band with your right hand
3. Extend your right arm up so the band is taut
4. Bring the arm back; repeat
5. Perform the exercise with the left hand on top

- Keep the lower elbow bent at a 90-degree position
- To make the exercise more difficult, pull the lower hand down

Banded Side Arm Raise
(Right, Left)

This exercise is great for strengthening your trapezius muscle and your side deltoids.

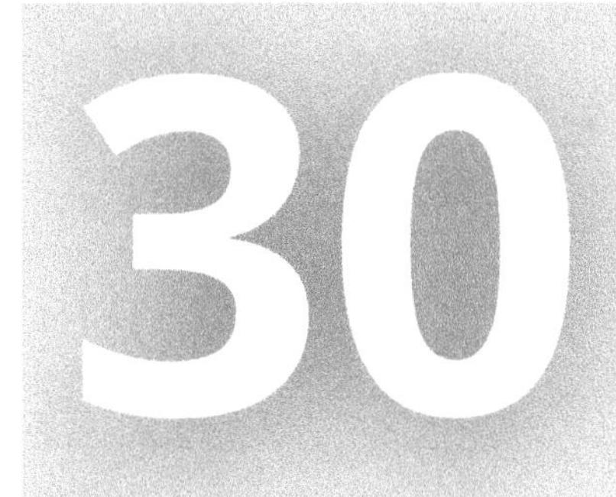

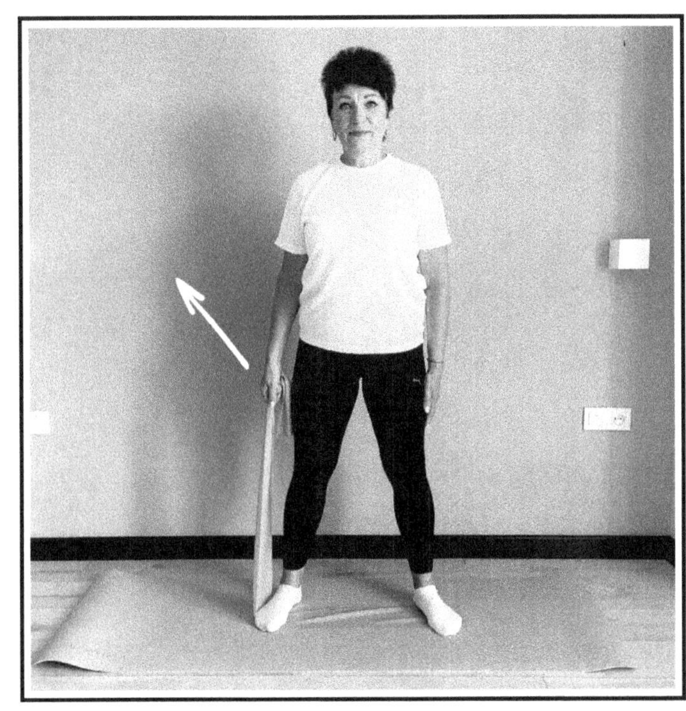 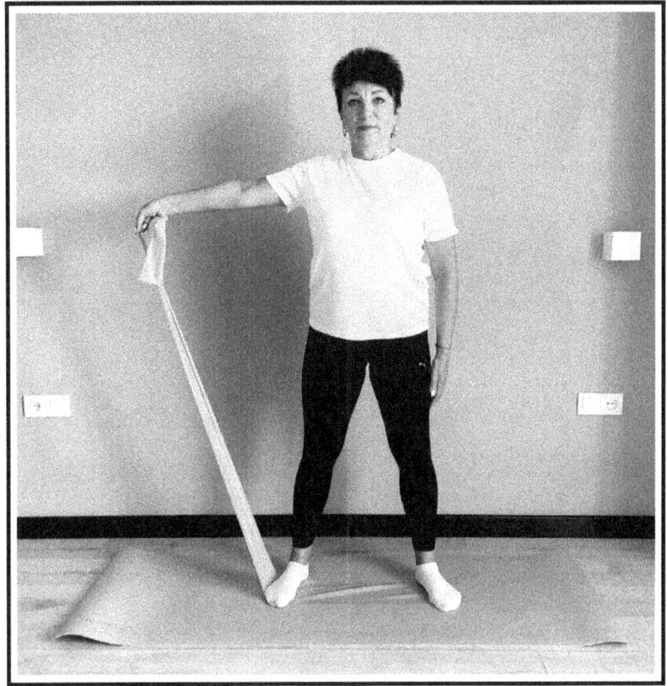

PROCEDURE:

1. Stand with two legs on one end of the band
2. Grab the other end with the right hand
3. Then lift your right arm sideways
4. Keep your right wrist and elbow in line with the shoulder
5. Bring the arm back; repeat
6. Perform the exercise with the left hand

SUGGESTED TIPS:

- Don't pull the band too high (not above shoulder level)
- Don't bend the arms
- At the beginning of the exercise, inhale; slowly exhale as you lift the arm up

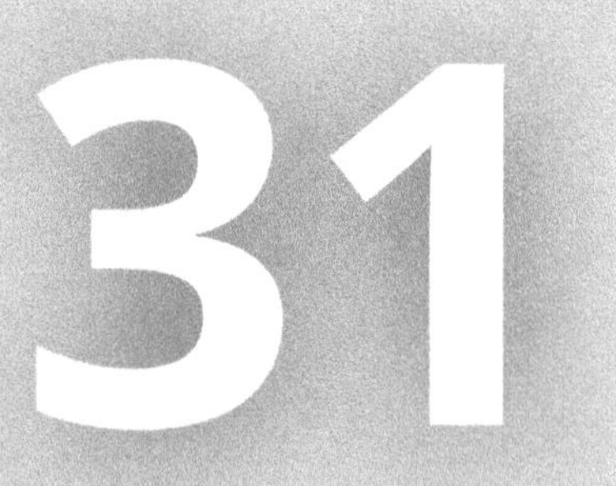

Ab Tilt

This exercise activates the core muscles (especially the abdominal muscles).

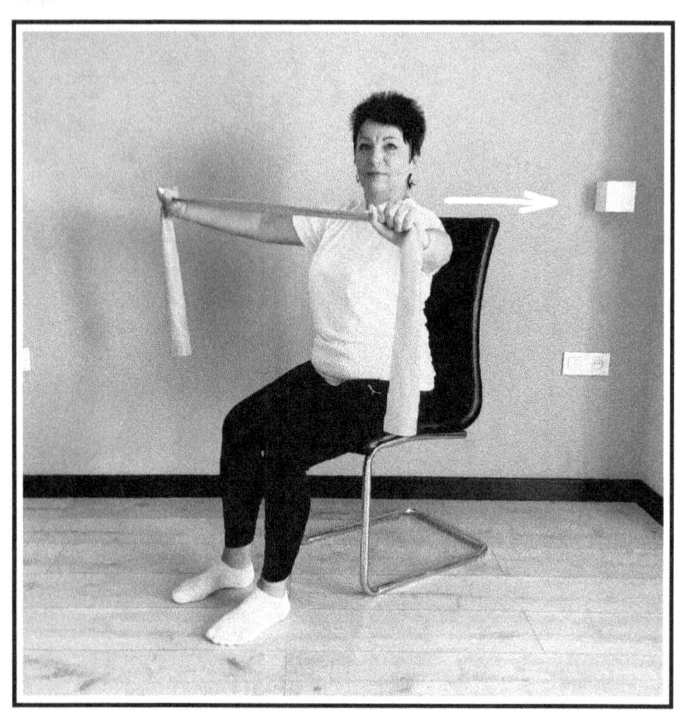

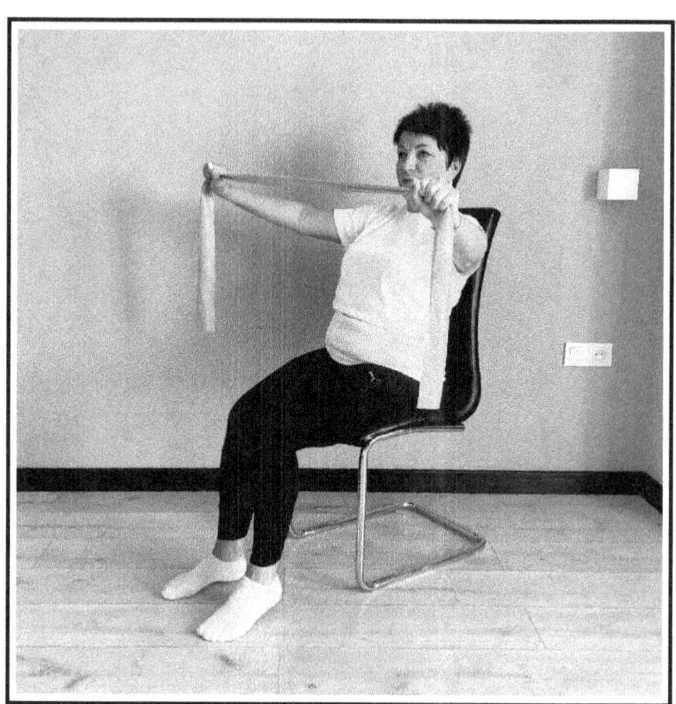

PROCEDURE:

1. Sit on a chair with your hands shoulder-width apart
2. Stretch the band in front of you
3. Engage your stomach muscles; lean slightly backward
4. Go back to the starting position
5. Repeat the movement

SUGGESTED TIPS:

- Don't rush the movement
- Engage the stomach muscles
- At the beginning of the movement, inhale; as you are leaning back, exhale

PAGE 50

Lower Body Exercises

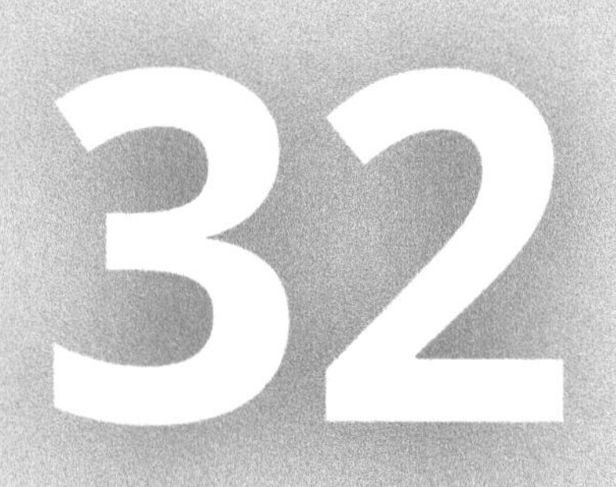

32

Band Resisted Glute Kicks
(Right, Left)

This is a great exercise to warm up your lower body while giving the glutes a lift.

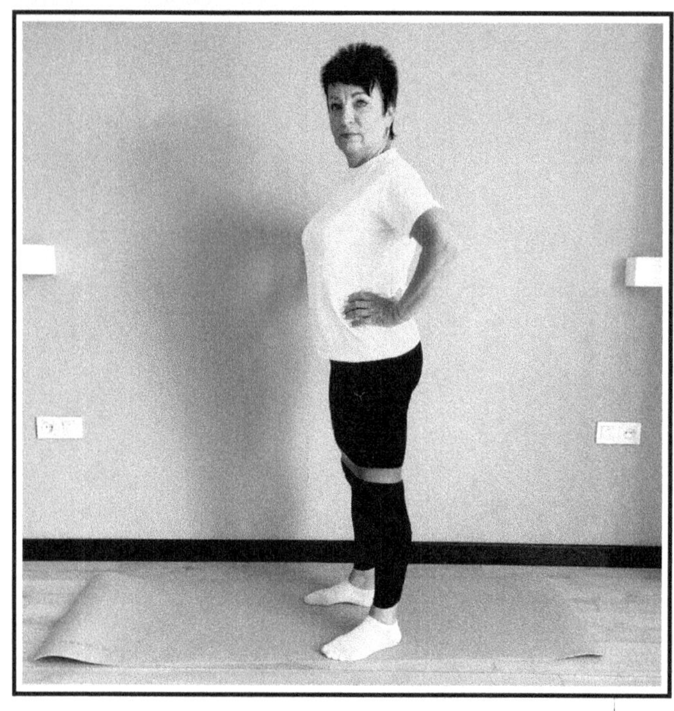

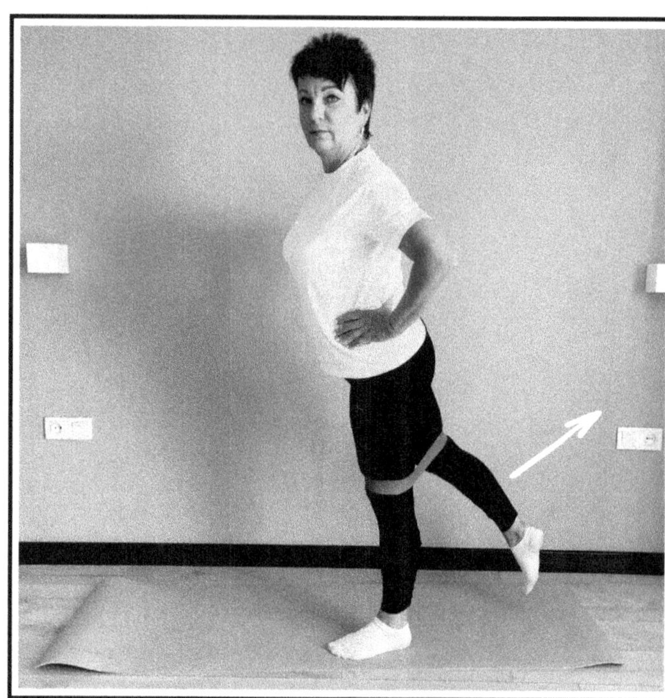

PROCEDURE:

1. Place a loop band around your legs above your knees
2. Kick your right leg directly behind you while pulling on the band
3. Repeat
4. Perform the exercise with the left leg

SUGGESTED TIPS:

- Don't use a band on bare skin (this can be especially painful if you have leg hair)
- Don't let the band slack; make sure to keep constant tension to achieve maximum resistance
- Keep your knee straight to concentrate on your glutes
- Move the band to your calves level for more resistance

Band Resistance Squats

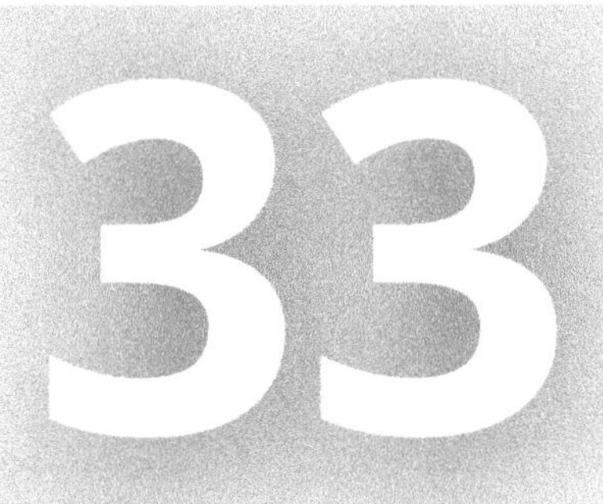

This squat helps shred your thighs and backside.

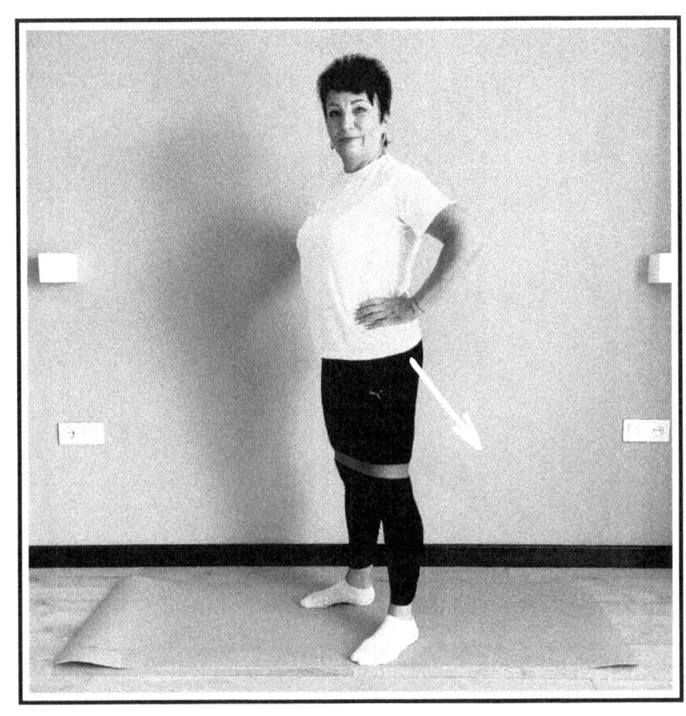 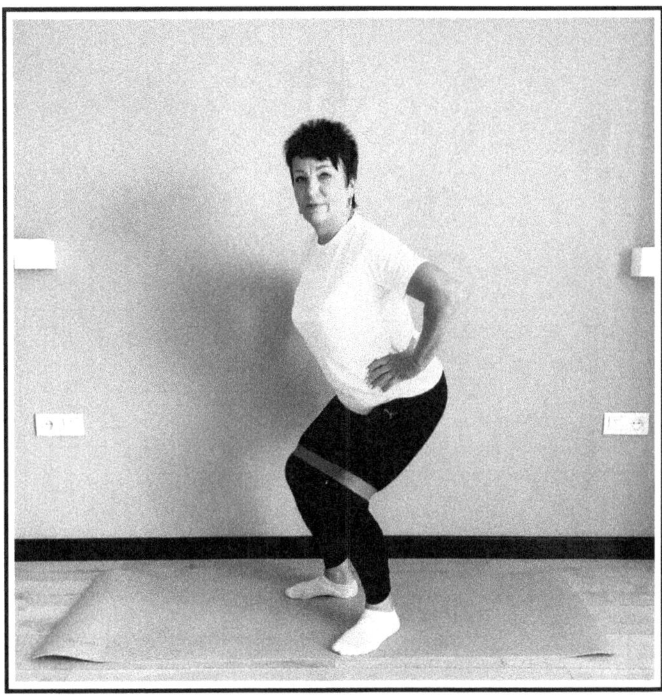

PROCEDURE:

1. Begin in a standing position; place a loop band around your legs right above the knee
2. Drop your hips toward the floor as you keep your heels on the floor
3. Go back up
4. Repeat the movement

SUGGESTED TIPS:

- Don't lean too far forward during the squat; sit back on your heels to target your hamstrings and glutes
- Keep the band from pulling your knees together; go deeper into the squat by pushing your knees apart

34 Banded Side Leg Raise
(Right, Left)

This exercise works on your gluteus medius muscle and also challenges your stability.

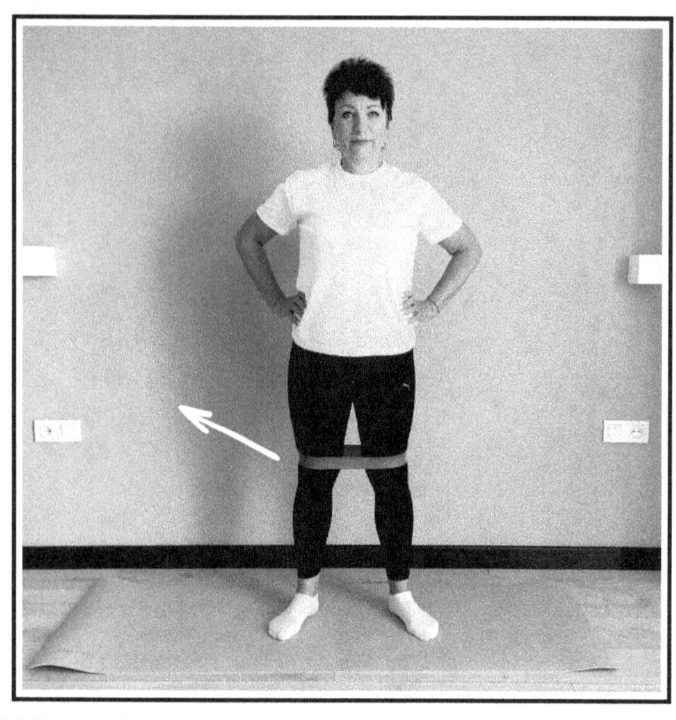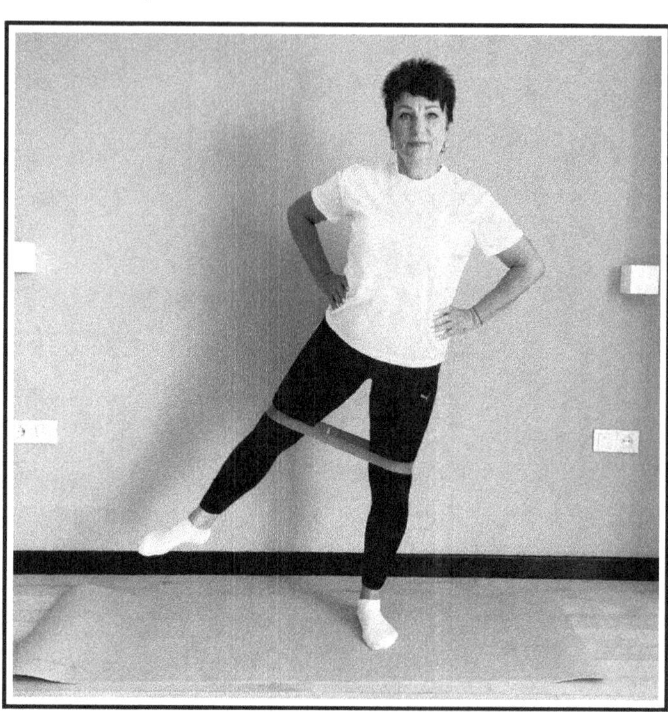

PROCEDURE:

1. Stand tall with your feet hip-width apart
2. Place a loop band around your legs right above the knees, keeping it taut
3. Lift your right leg to the side; bring it back
4. Repeat the movement
5. Perform the exercise using the left leg

SUGGESTED TIPS:

- Don't hold the breath
- Hold onto a chair or stand next to the wall to make the exercise easier

PAGE 54

Banded Windshield Wiper (Right, Left)

This exercise helps reduce your lower back stiffness.

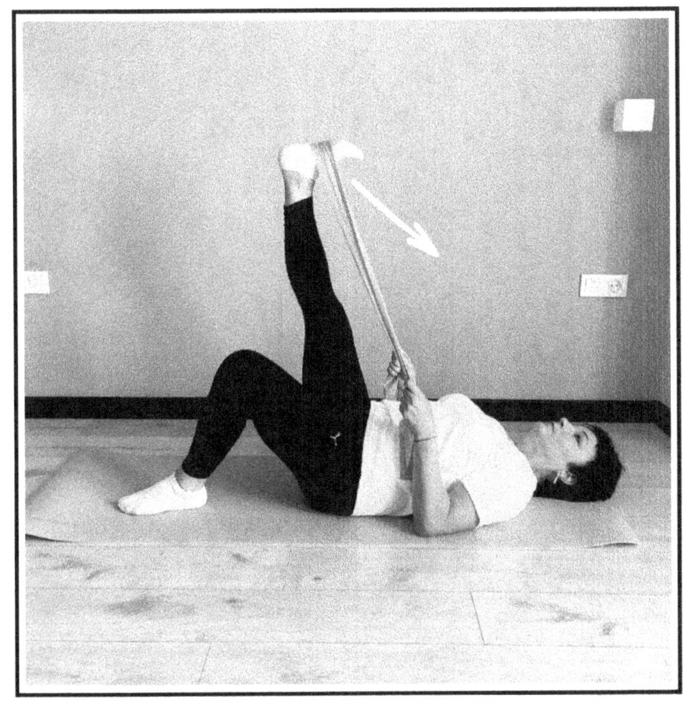
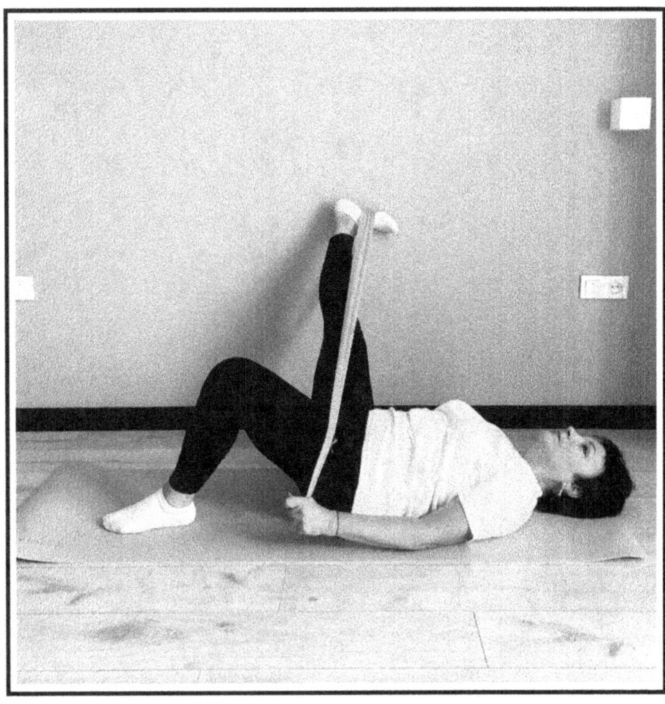

PROCEDURE:

1. Lie on the floor; have the band looped around your right foot, grabbing the ends
2. Lift your right leg upward to the ceiling
3. Lower your extended leg to the right side
4. Return it back; repeat the movement
5. Perform the exercise using the left leg

SUGGESTED TIPS:

- Don't bend your extended leg
- Don't rush the movement
- Concentrate on your breathing
- Slowly perform the movement

36 Banded Knee Raises
(Right, Left)

This is a lower-body movement that can improve your hip mobility and balance.

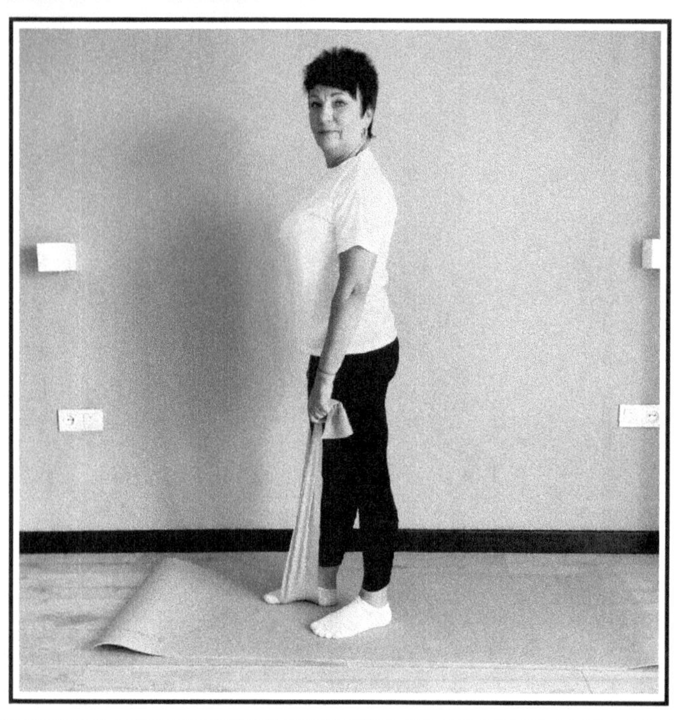 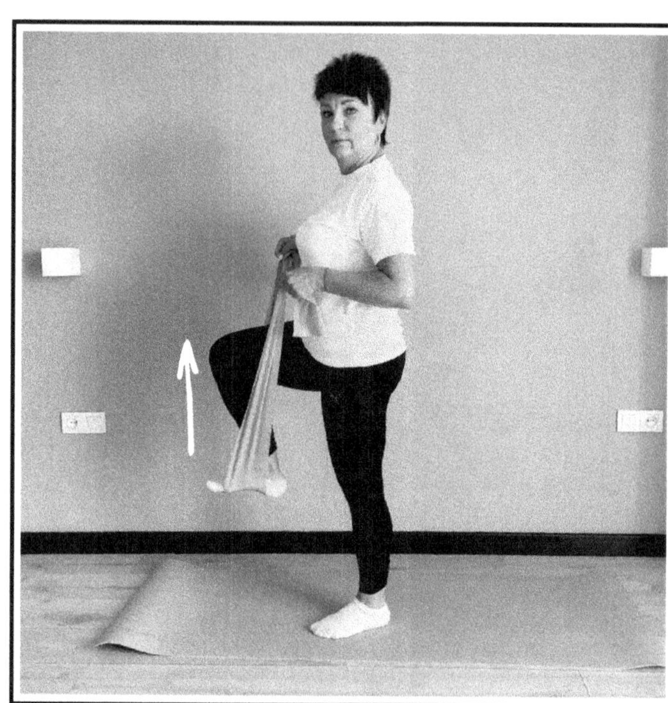

PROCEDURE:

1. Stand tall with feet shoulder-width apart; loop a band under your right foot
2. Lift your right knee with your hands at your waist level, keeping the band taut
3. Push your right knee down
4. Repeat the movement
5. Perform the exercise using the other leg

SUGGESTED TIPS:

- Don't rush the movement
- Don't hold the breath
- Squeeze the floor with your foot that's on the floor to improve your balance

PAGE 56

Banded Donkey Kicks
(Right, Left)

This exercise will set your butt on fire while challenging your stability and working your entire leg.

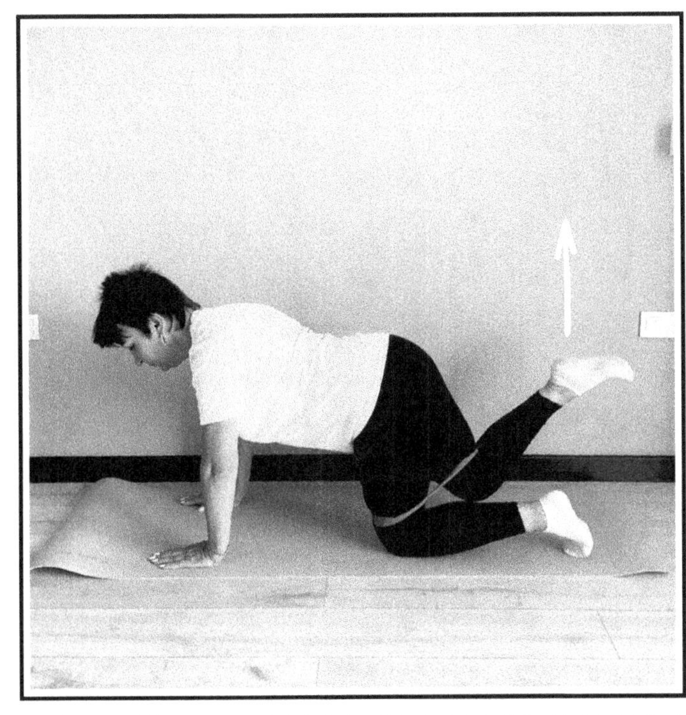

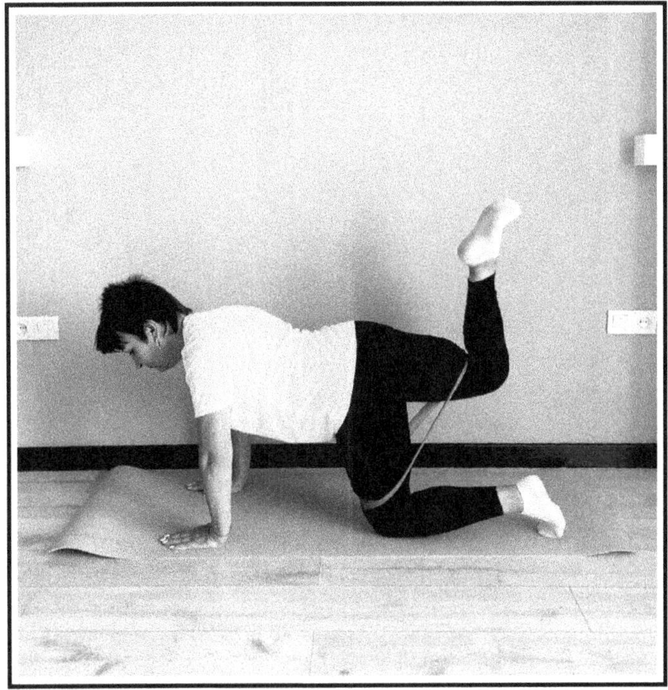

1. Get on all fours; place your hands directly under your shoulders and your knees under your hips
2. Place a loop loop band around your legs right above the knees, keeping it taut
3. Slowly lift your leg straight back and up toward the ceiling while keeping a 90-degree bend in your right knee
4. Bring the leg down; repeat
5. Perform the exercise using the left leg

SUGGESTED TIPS:

- Don't arch the lower back
- Don't rotate your hips to one side as you raise the working leg
- Perform the move in full range of motion; engage the core and breathe throughout the exercise

38 Lying Leg Lifts
(Right, Left)

This exercise is a great fit for stretching hamstrings, calves, and glute muscles.

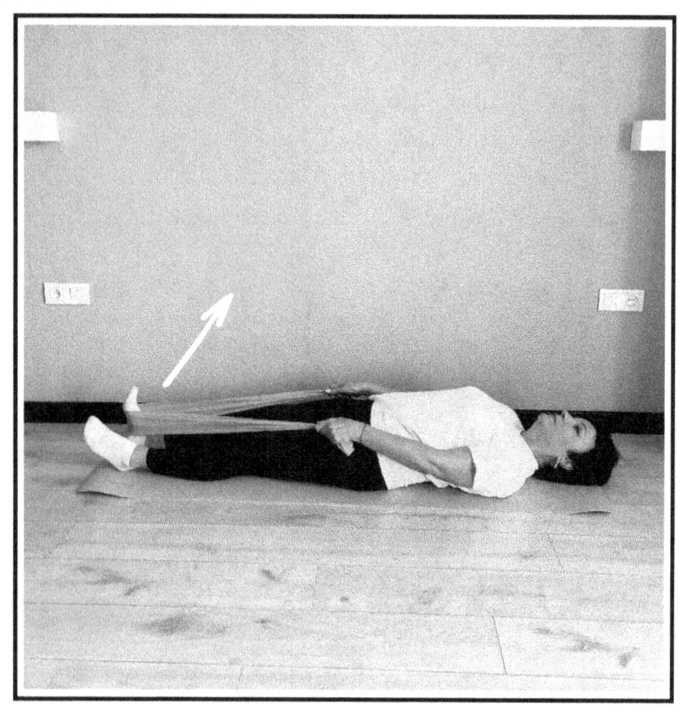

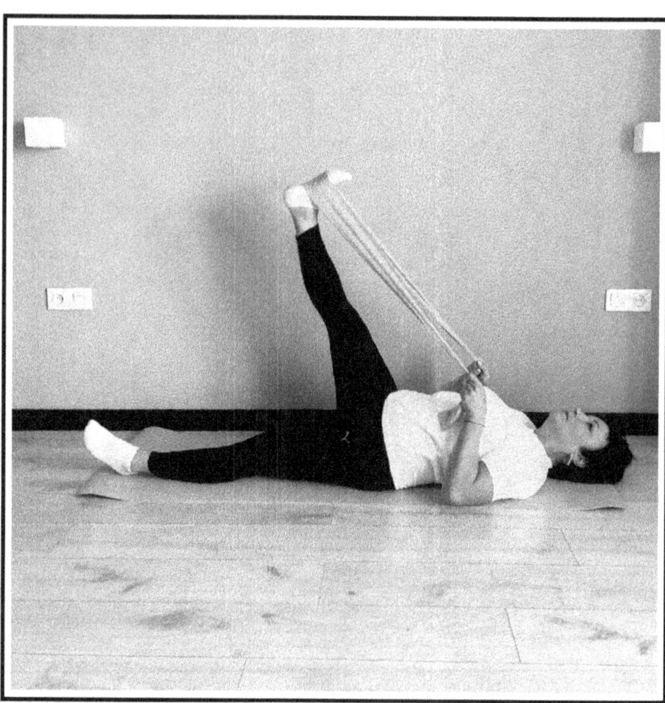

1. Lie on the floor extending your legs; have the band looped around your right foot, grabbing the ends
2. Extend your right leg up bringing your hands to your chest; slowly lower your leg down
3. Repeat the movement
4. Perform the exercise using the left leg

SUGGESTED TIPS:

- Don't rush the movement
- Don't bend the leg
- Maintain a steady breathing pattern throughout this movement

Banded Leg Press
(Right, Left)

Banded leg presses work your quadriceps and glute muscles.

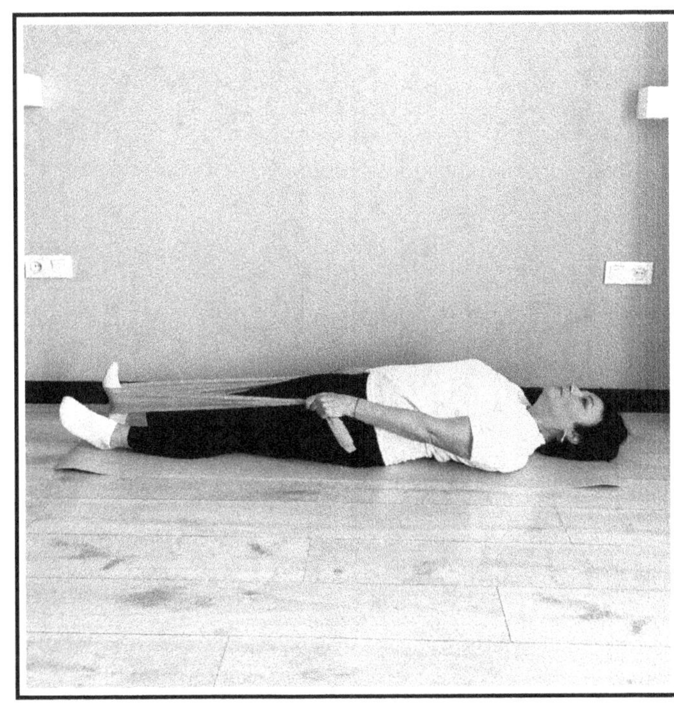
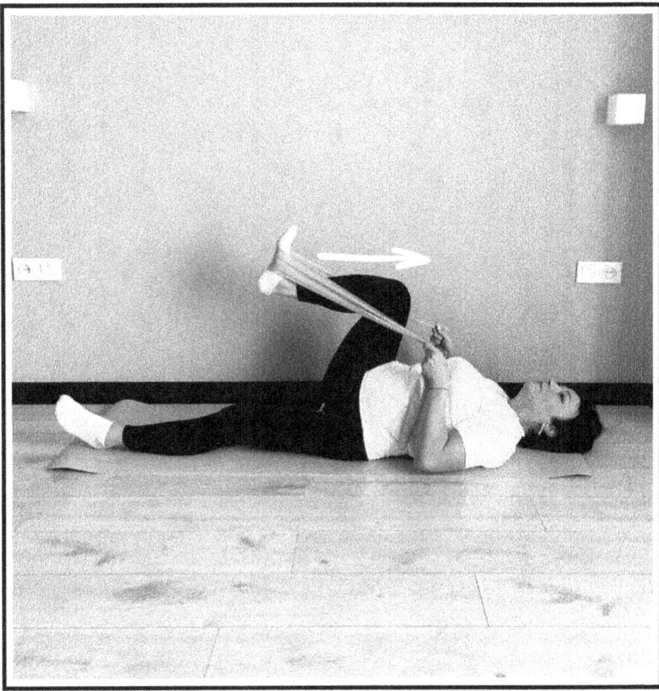

PROCEDURE:

1. Lay on your back with the lower back touching the floor
2. Loop the band around your right foot
3. Lift your right leg and push it forward while resisting the band with your hands
4. Bring the leg back; repeat the movement
5. Perform the exercise using the left leg

SUGGESTED TIPS:

- Pull and resist the band with your hands
- Don't go too fast
- Start with the weakest band and increase the difficulty with other bands as you progress on this exercise

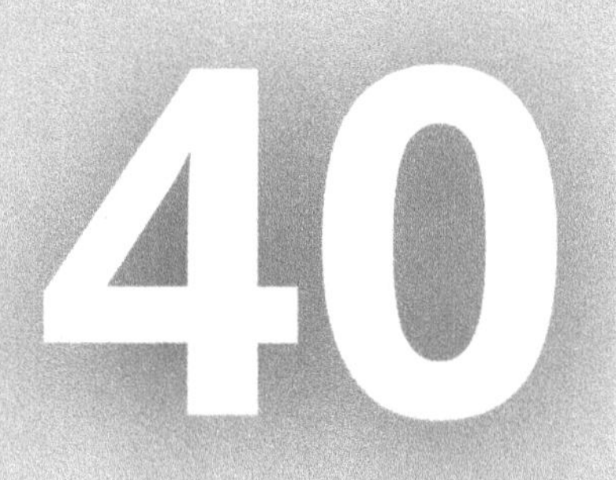

Banded Glute Bridge

This exercise tones your thighs and pumps up your glutes to make your lower body look perfect.

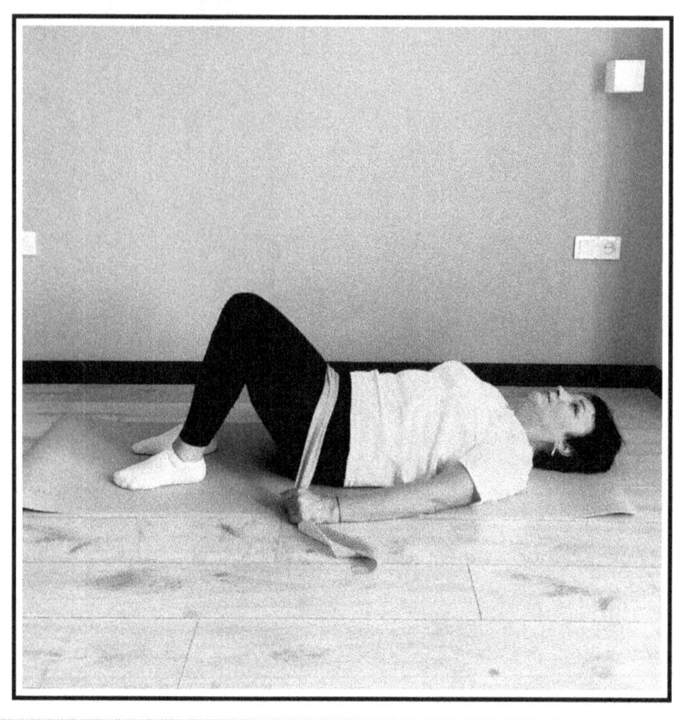 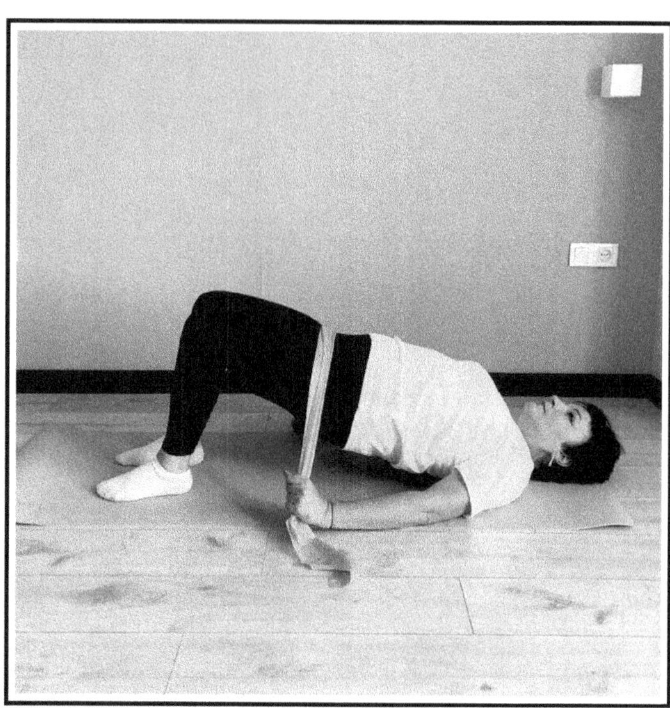

PROCEDURE:

1. Lie down on the back; bend your knees
2. For added resistance, wrap a band above your pelvic area and hold the ends with your hands
3. Raise your hips and squeeze your glutes; your heels and shoulders should be on the floor
4. In a controlled movement, lower the hips to the starting position
5. Repeat the movement

SUGGESTED TIPS:

- Don't put your heels too far out, so that the glute bridge is too low
- Don't let your glutes rest; strain them even when your hips are down

Banded Squat With Abduction (Right, Left)

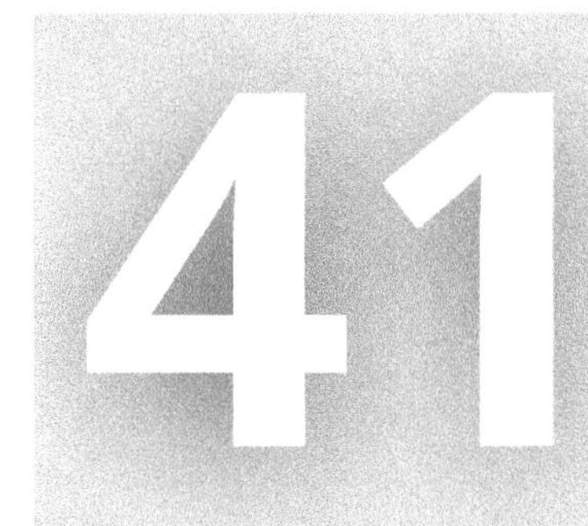

This single-leg squat with hip abduction works the legs, abdominals, hips, and buttocks.

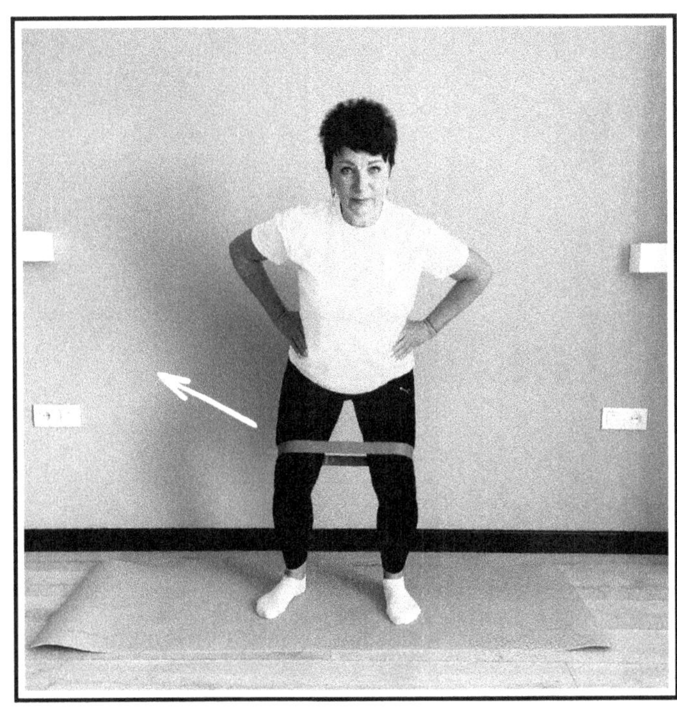
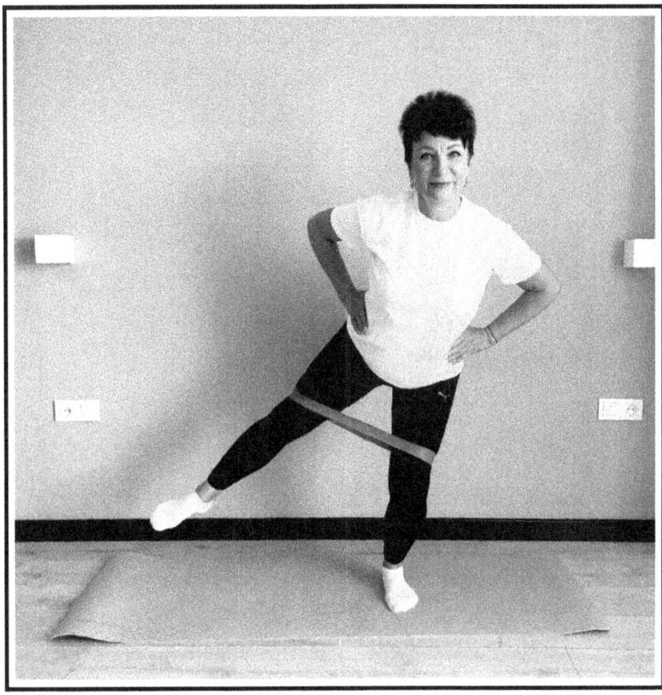

PROCEDURE:

1. Stand up straight with your feet shoulder-width apart; wrap a loop band around your knees
2. Bend your knees slightly; lift your right hip to the side while balancing on your left foot
3. Lower your right knee down and repeat the movement
4. Perform the exercise using the other leg

SUGGESTED TIPS:

- Don't round your back
- Don't balance on your toes
- Hold your chest high with your knees pushed out while balancing on your whole foot

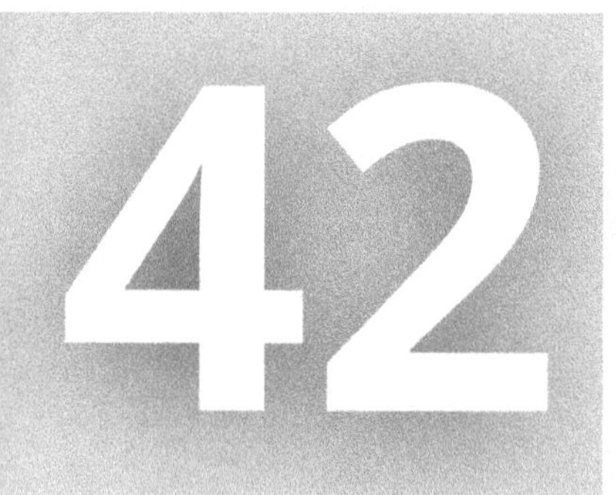

42 Banded Leg Extensions
(Right, Left)

This exercise will set your butt on fire while challenging your stability and also working your entire leg.

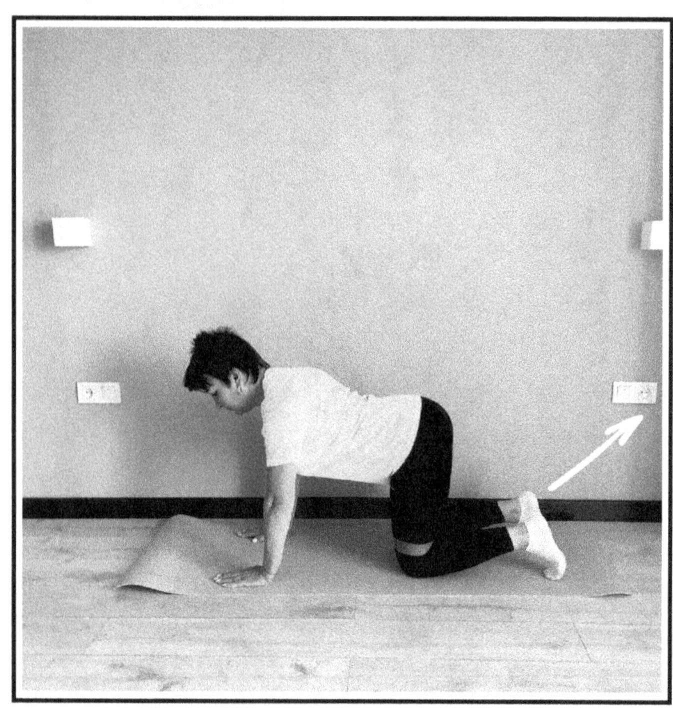
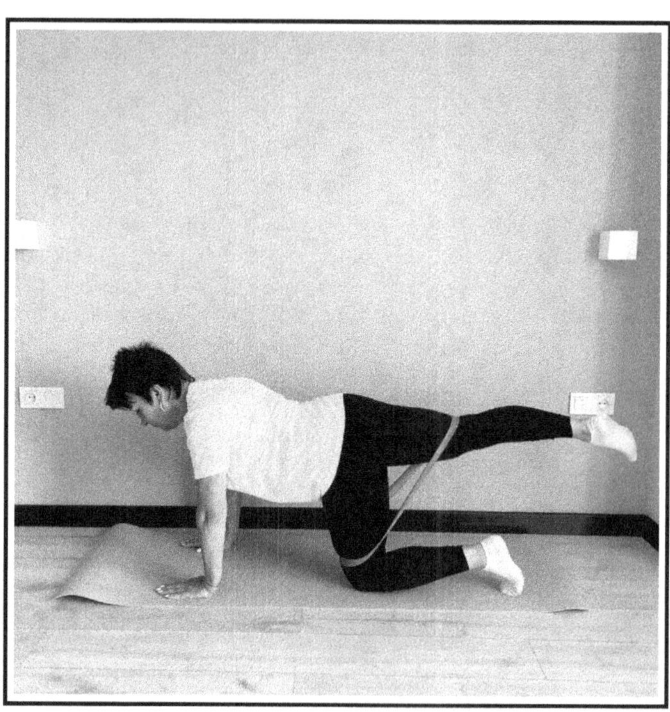

PROCEDURE:

1. Get on all fours; place your hands directly under your shoulders and your knees under your hips
2. Place a loop band around your legs right above the knees, keeping it taut; extend your right leg up and backward
3. Bring the leg back and repeat the movement
4. Perform the exercise using the other leg

SUGGESTED TIPS:

- Don't arch the lower back
- Don't rotate your hips to one side as you raise the working leg
- Perform the move in the full range of motion; engage the core and breathe throughout the exercise
- If you have trouble keeping your balance, lean your side against the wall

Banded Glute Bridge

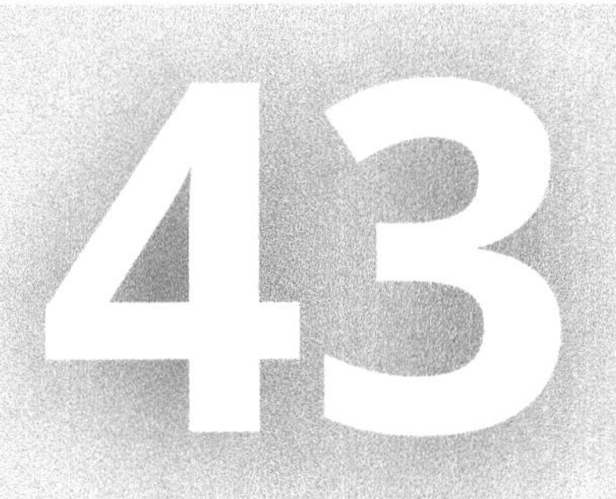

This exercise is great for preventing and rehabilitating knee and back injuries.

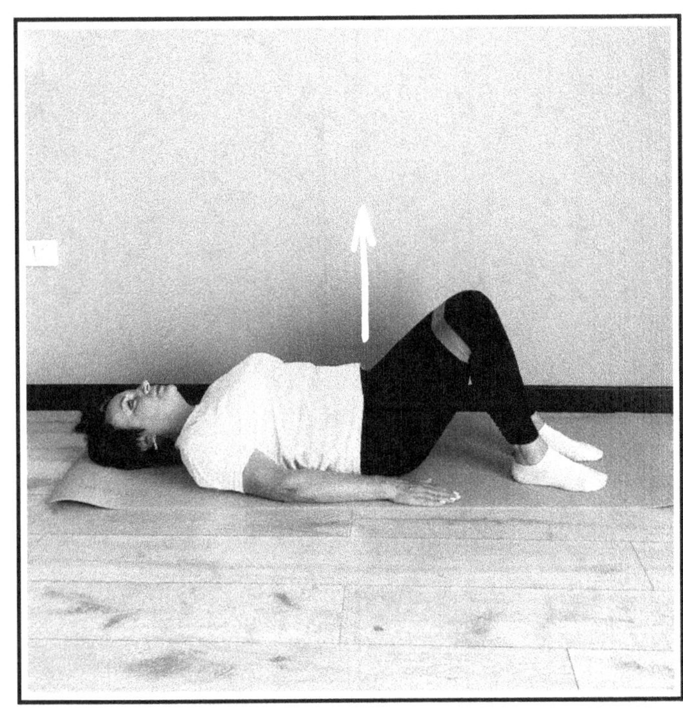
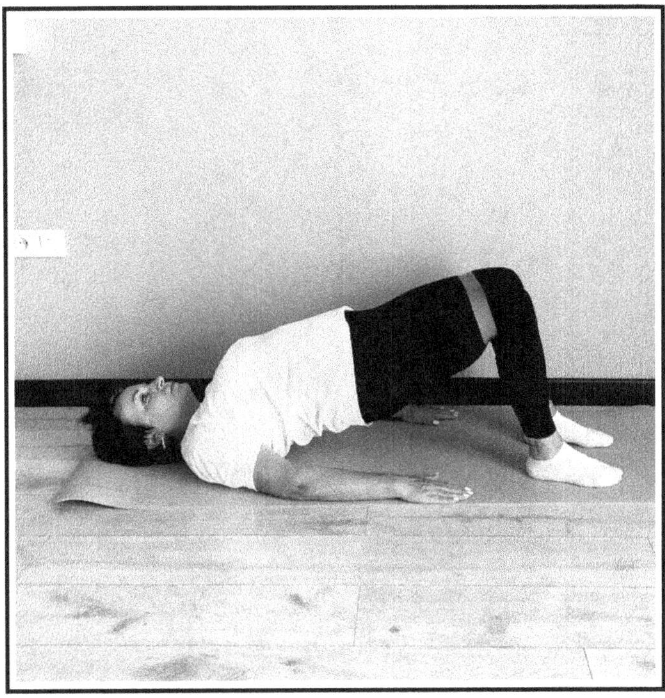

PROCEDURE:

1. Lie down on the floor; have your back straight against the floor with your knees at right angles
2. Place a loop band around both thighs to rest right above your knees
3. Keep your arms down at your side with your knees pressed out against the band; raise your hips toward the ceiling
4. Squeeze your muscles tight and hold for 2-3 seconds, then release; go down; repeat

SUGGESTED TIPS:

- Don't have your hips too low or too high
- Don't bend your lower back
- Don't cave your knees in toward one another
- Keep your glutes and spine tight with your knees pushed outward

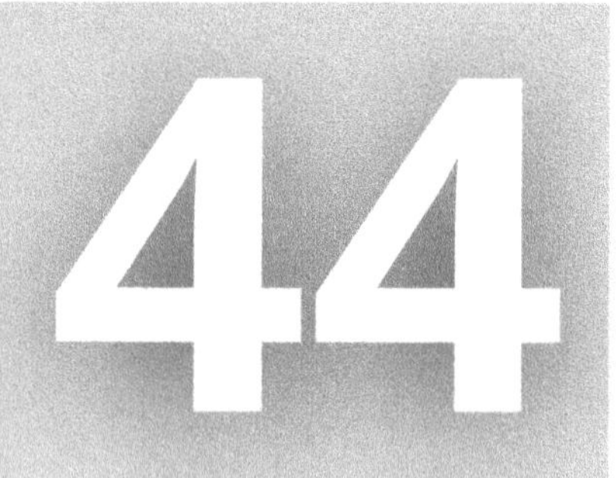

44 Single Leg Hip Abduction
(Right, Left)

This exercise is great for engaging the glutes.

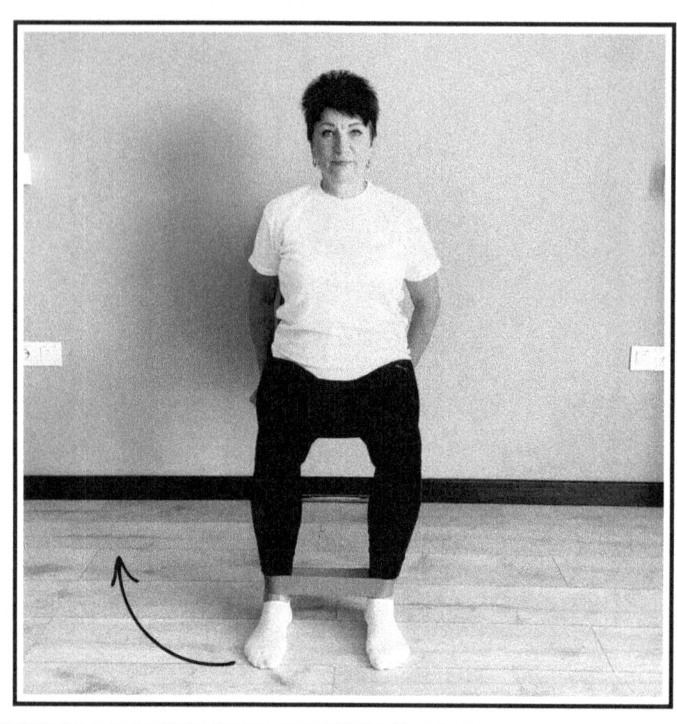

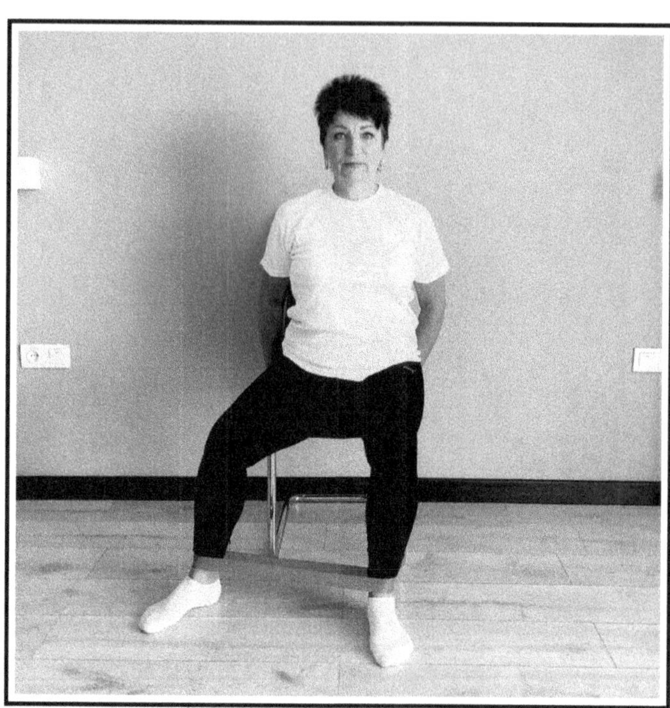

PROCEDURE:

1. To start, sit on a chair with your knees bent
2. With your knees hip-width apart, wrap a loop band slightly above your ankles
3. In a controlled motion, slowly push your right knee out to the side and then bring it back; repeat
4. Perform the exercise on the left side

SUGGESTED TIPS:

- Don't have your feet too close
- Don't do a short-range movement
- Keep your core tight
- Hold your head up, face forward; maintain an upright posture throughout the exercise
- Don't rush the exercise

Banded-Feet Activation
(Right, Left)

This is a great exercise for strengthening and stretching your calf muscles. It's also great for keeping the ankles healthy by working your plantar and dorsal flexion of the ankle joint.

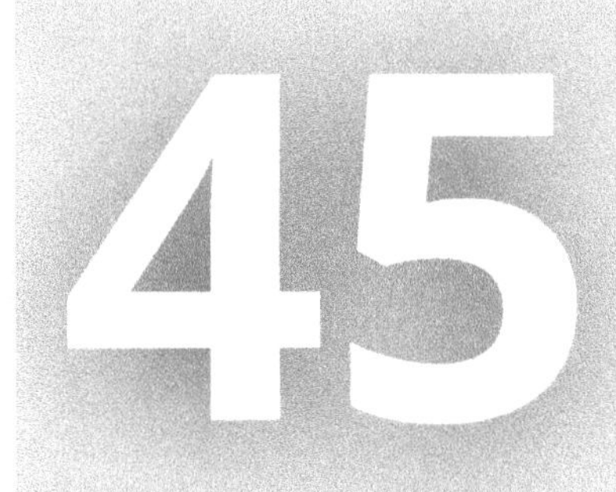

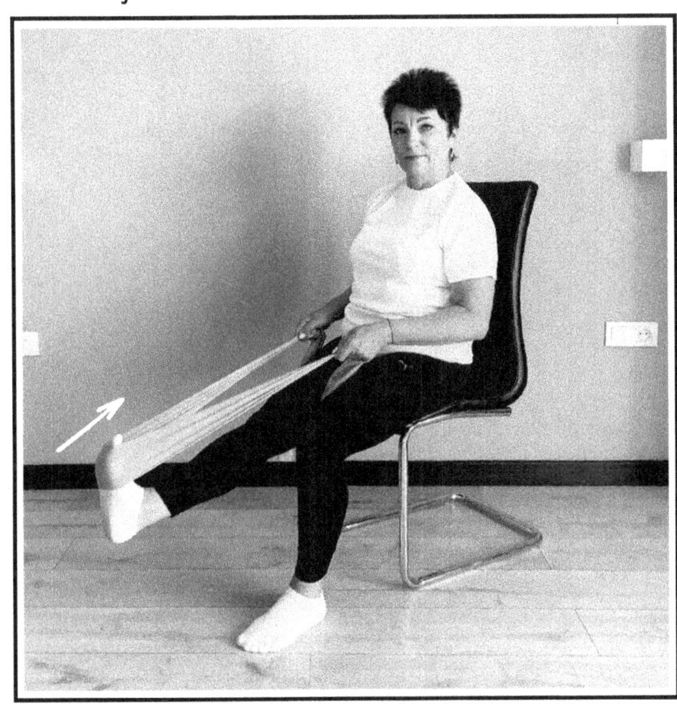

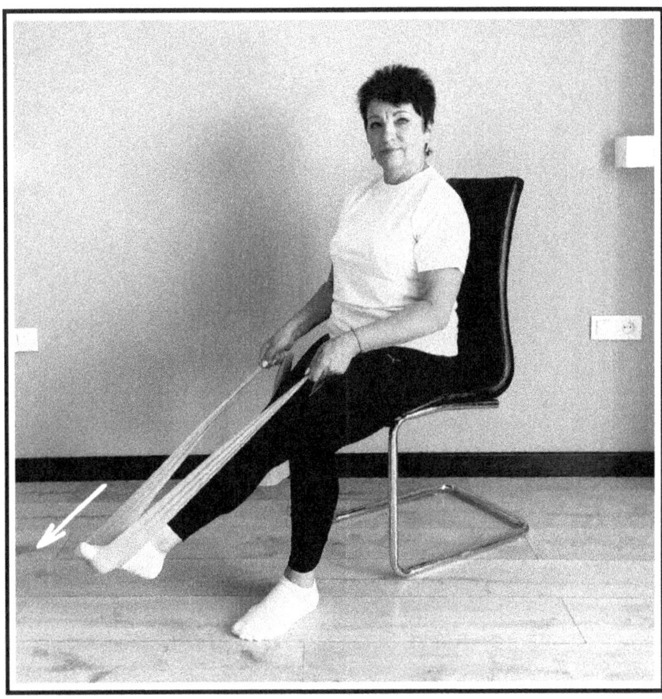

PROCEDURE:

1. Sit straight on a chair
2. Extend your right leg and loop the band under your toes
3. Stretch the band with your hands and move your toes up and down
4. Perform the exercise with the other leg

SUGGESTED TIPS:

- Don't go too fast
- Don't round the back

Banded Hip Raises

This exercise strengthens your hip flexors which tend to weaken from different lifestyle habits.

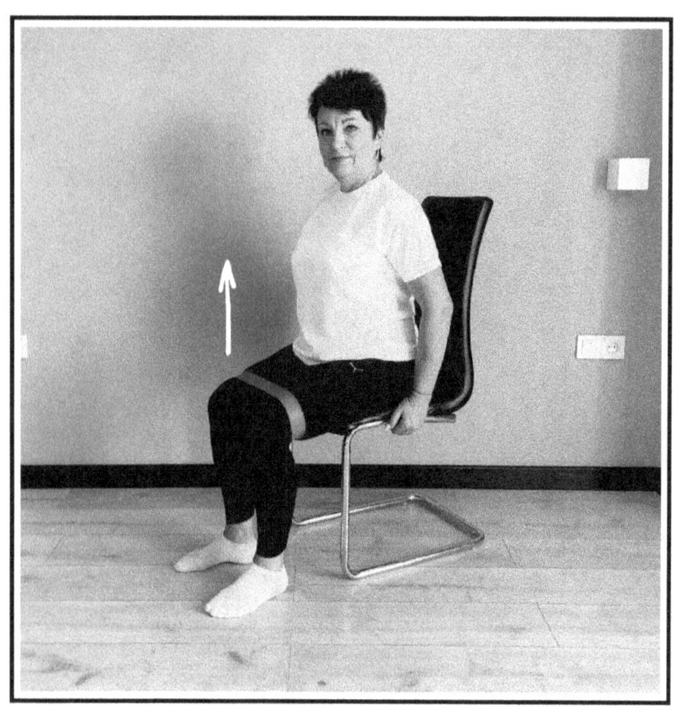 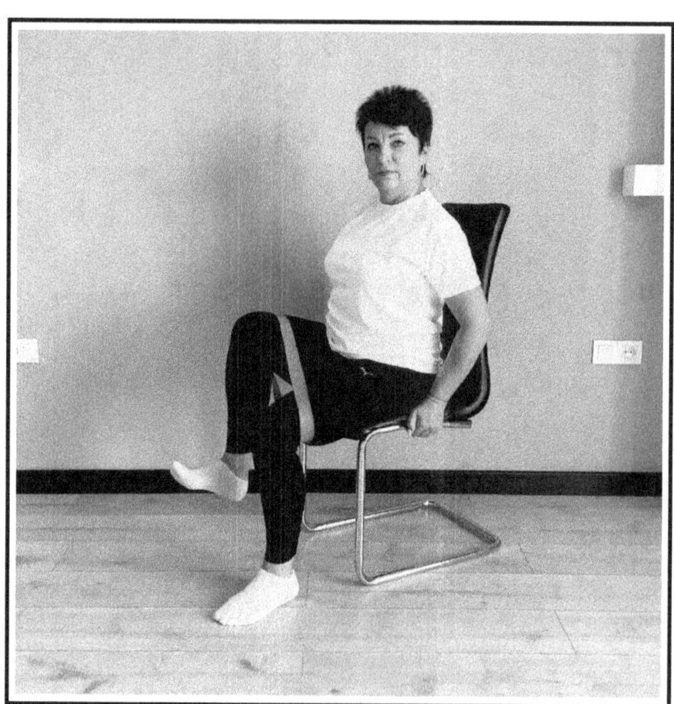

PROCEDURE:

1. Sit on a chair with your feet hip-width apart
2. Loop the band above your knees
3. Lift one leg and hold it for one second
4. Bring the leg back
5. Alternate between legs

SUGGESTED TIPS:

- Don't go too fast
- Start with the weakest band and increase the difficulty with other bands as you progress on this exercise

Banded Duck Walks
(Forward, Backward)

This is a good exercise to activate your entire lower body.

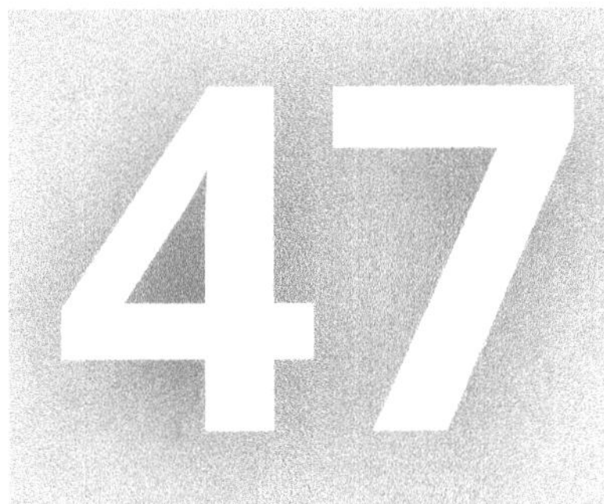
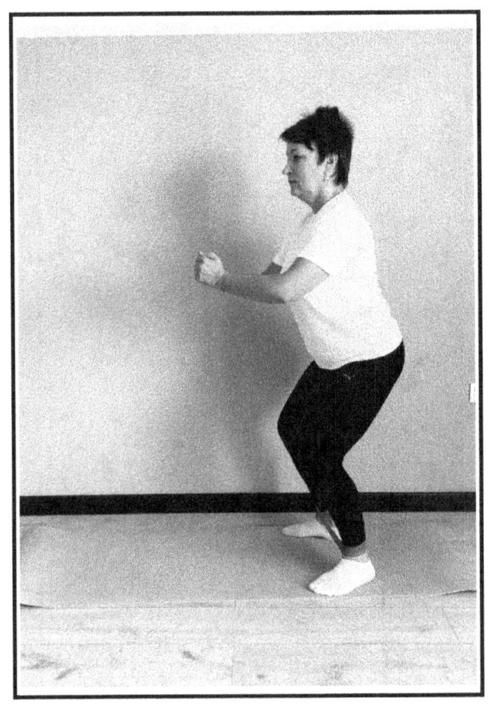
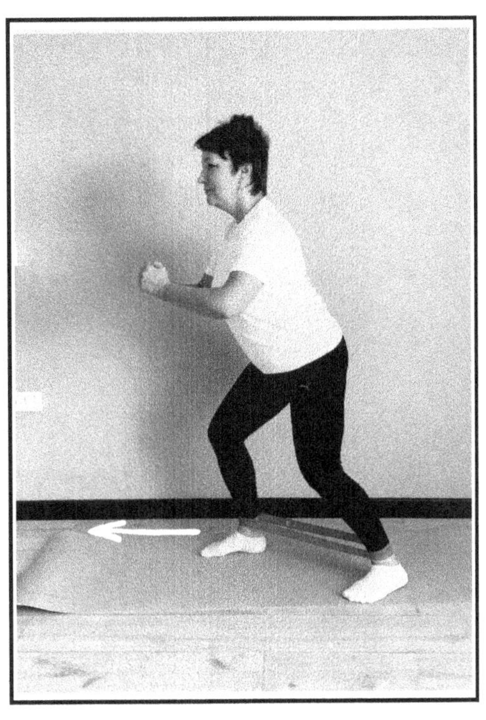
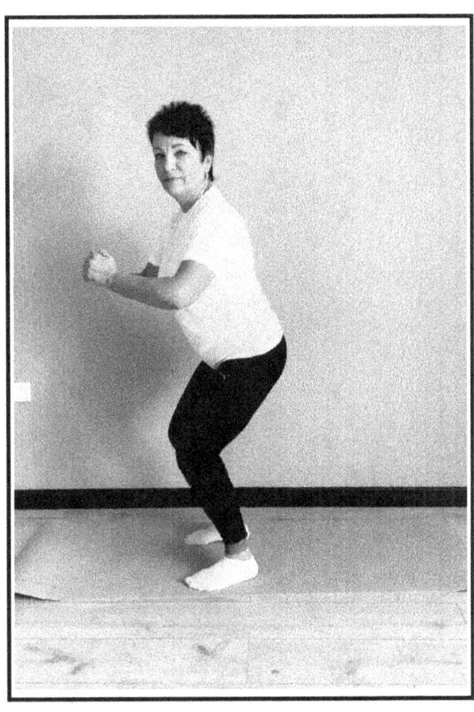

PROCEDURE:

1. Start in a half-squat position with the loop band around your ankles
2. Walk a few steps forward while keeping tension on the band, then walk backward to your starting position
3. Repeat

SUGGESTED TIPS:

- Don't let the band slack; make sure to keep constant tension to achieve maximum resistance
- Start with your feet wider apart and take bigger steps to increase the resistance for a more challenging workout

48

Seated Hip Abduction

Seated hip abductions work your gluteus medius muscle.

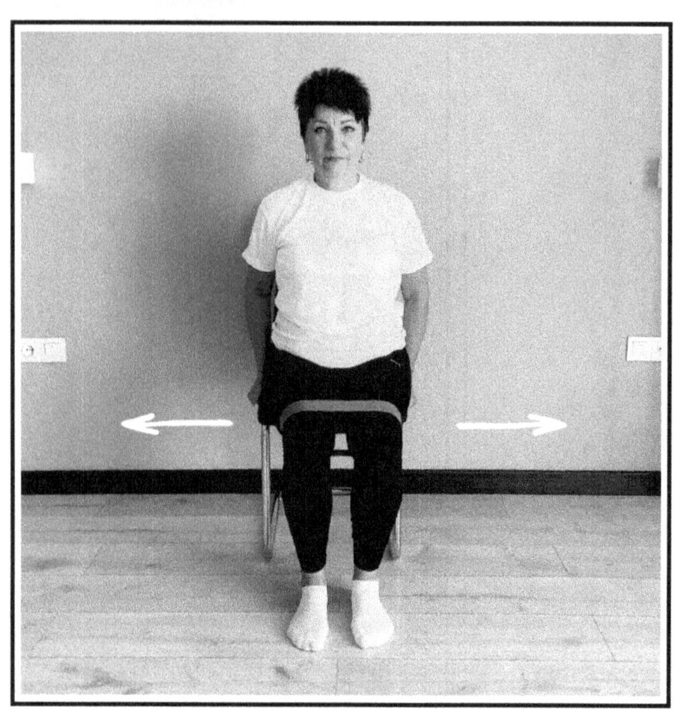 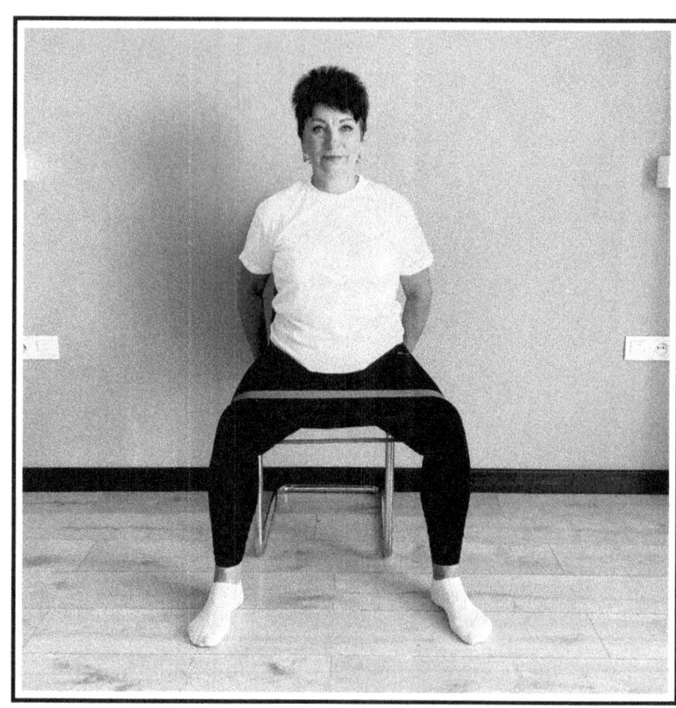

1. Sit tall on a chair
2. Have the hip band looped around your legs above your knees
3. Put your feet together
4. Then move your knees and feet to the side as far as you can
5. Go back slowly to the starting position
6. Repeat the movement

SUGGESTED TIPS:

- Don't rush the movement
- Don't hold the breath
- Adjust the difficulty of this exercise by using lighter or stronger bands

PAGE 68

Banded Side-to-Side Walk

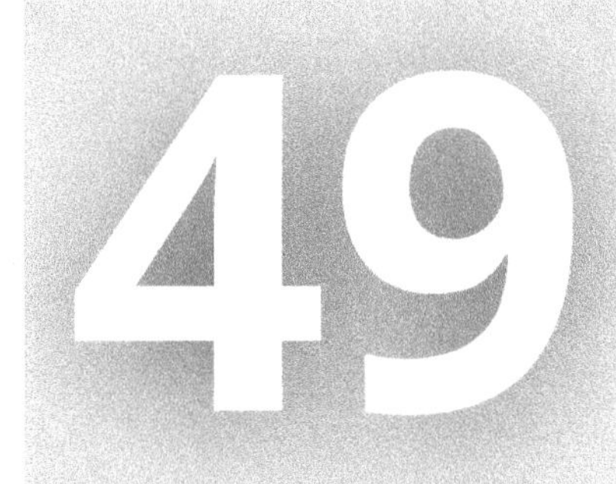

This exercise is a great way to quickly warm up the lower body while toning your backside and thighs.

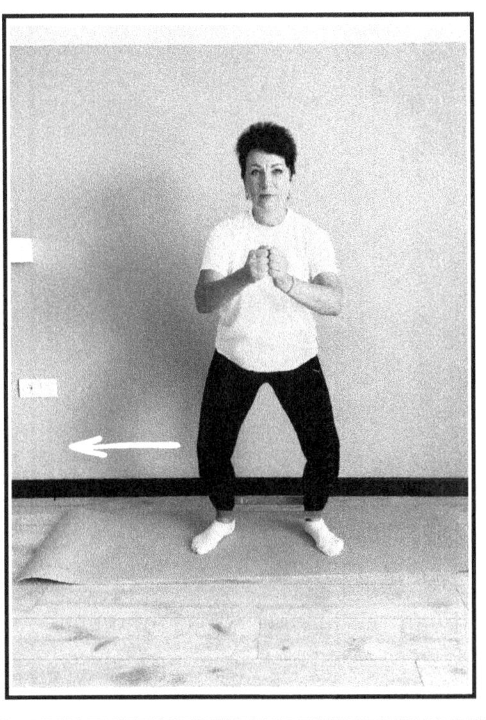 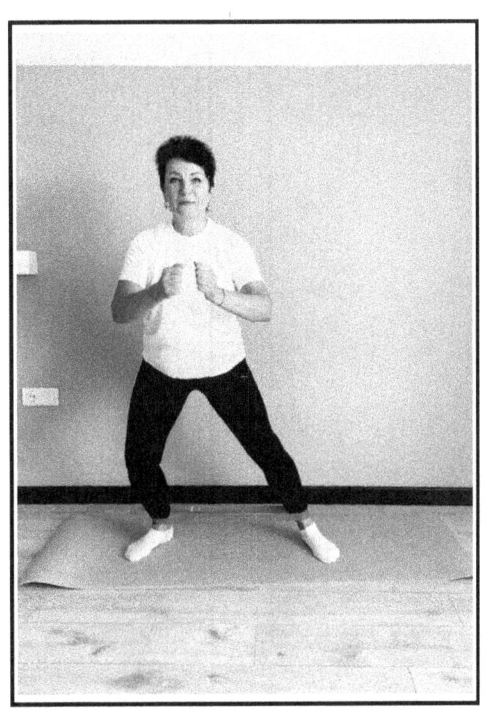 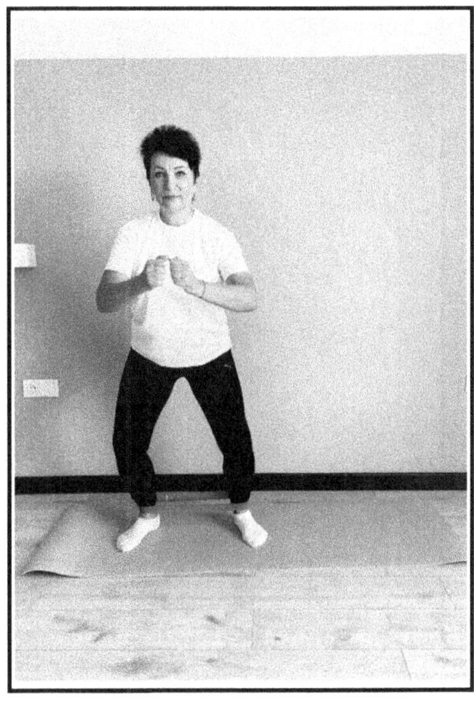

PROCEDURE:

1. Stand with your knees slightly bent and your butt back; keep your body slightly tilted forward
2. Place a loop band around your legs at ankle height
3. Walk two steps to the left, then take two steps to the right
4. Repeat

SUGGESTED TIPS:

- Add resistance if the movement is too easy (start with your legs further apart and keep more distance between them as you walk)

Banded Hip Flexors March Supine

This exercise targets the muscles in your hip flexors while utilizing the abdominal muscles to perform the movement.

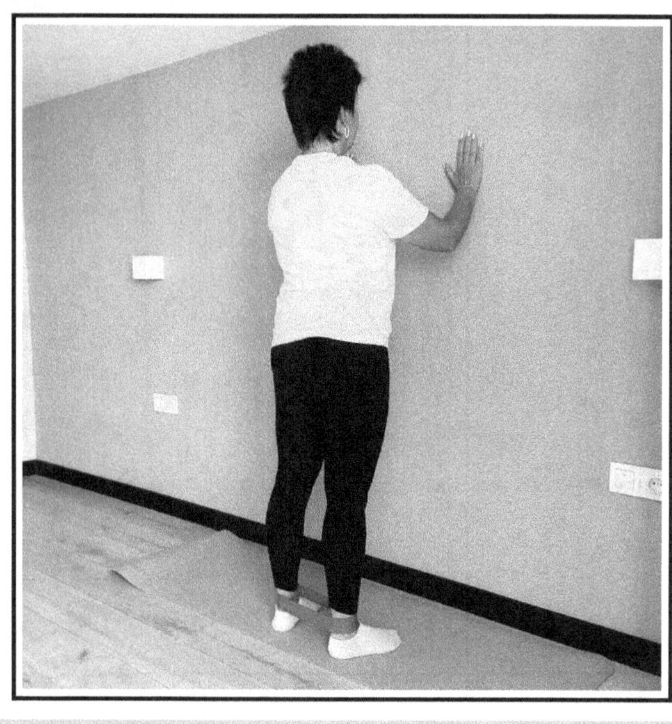
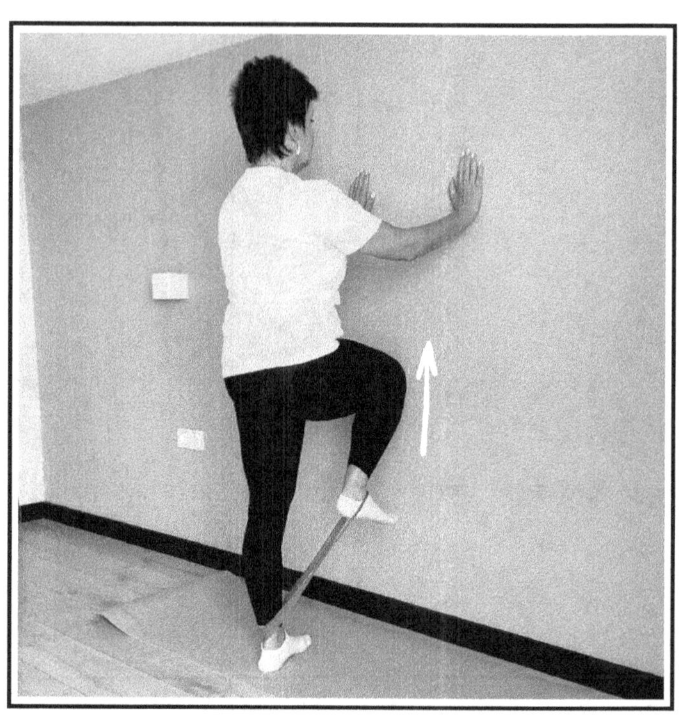

PROCEDURE:

1. Stand facing a wall with your palms touching it
2. Have your hip distance apart; keep your chest lifted and core engaged
3. Place a loop band around the balls of both feet
4. Contract your abdominal muscles; bring your left knee up and out in front of you (like you are marching); stop when the knee reaches the height of your hips
5. Return to starting position; alternate between legs

SUGGESTED TIPS:

- Don't round or dip your lower back
- Engage the core muscles
- Squeeze your hips to reach a neutral back position; keep the core tight

PAGE 70

Band Resisted Knees to Chest

This exercise fires up your abdominal muscles while improving stability and taking your endurance to the next level.

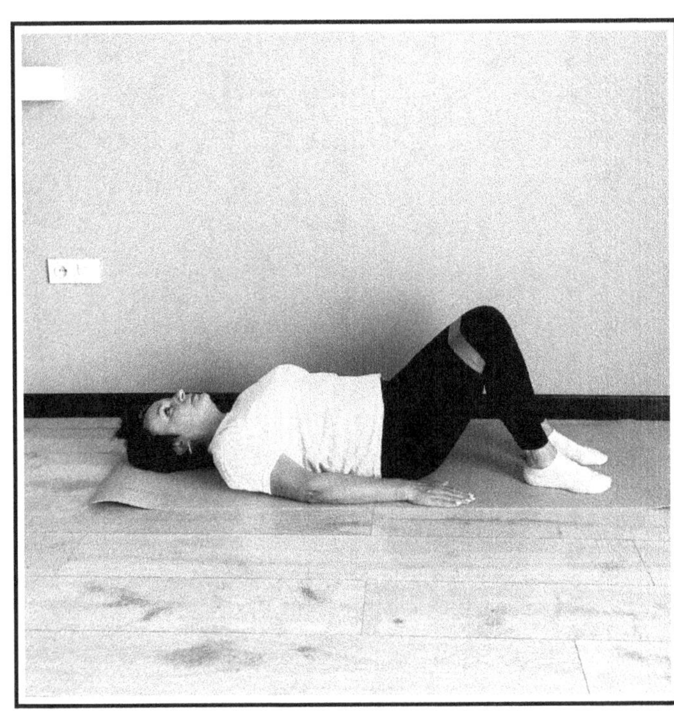 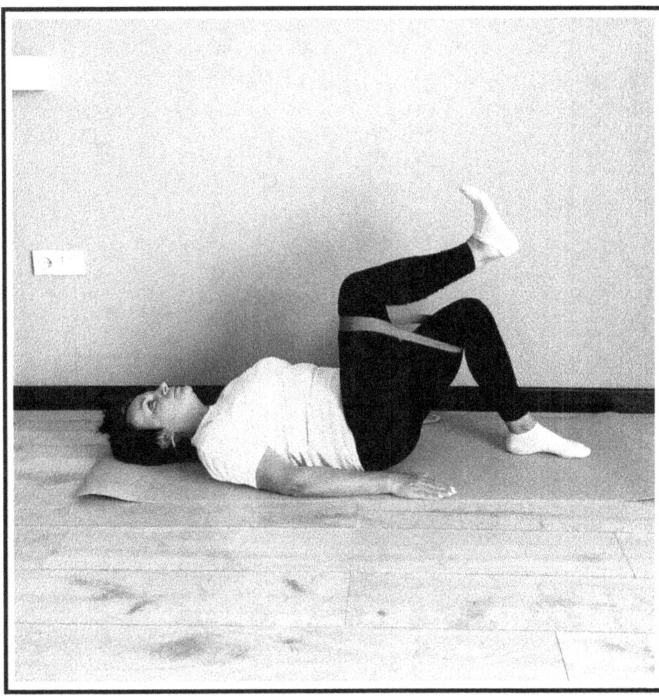

1. Lie down on the back; bend your knees
2. Place a loop band around your legs right above the knees, keeping it taut
3. Lift your right leg to your chest; don't straighten the leg and keep a 90-degree angle while lifting
4. Bring the right leg back; repeat alternating legs

- Don't switch legs too fast
- Make sure to brace your core
- Keep your head and shoulders on the floor to avoid overstraining your neck

Stretches

Tricep Stretch with a Band
(Right, Left)

This is a great exercise for stretching your triceps muscles and working your internal shoulder rotation.

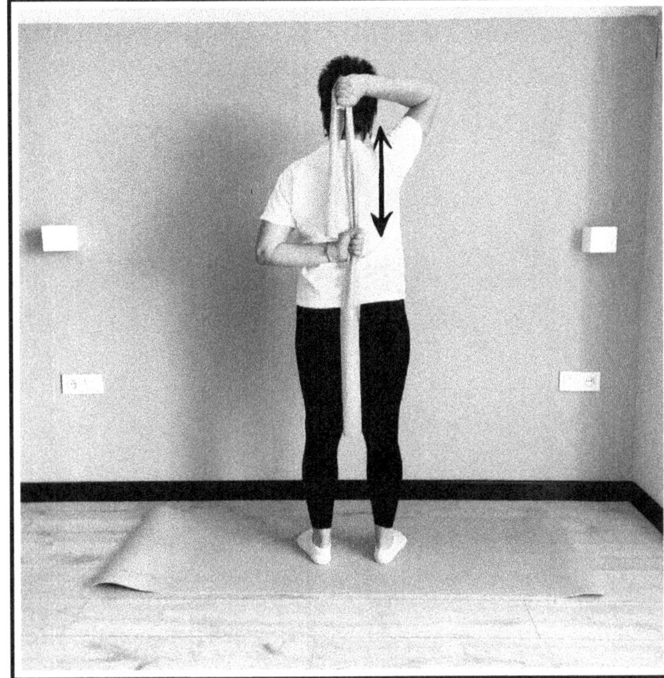

1. Stand tall and hold the band behind your back
2. Grab the bottom of the band with your left hand and the top of the band with your right hand
3. Gently stretch the band down with your left hand; hold the static stretch
4. Perform the same exercise with the other hand

SUGGESTED TIPS:

- Don't hold the breath
- To make the exercise more difficult, use a variety of resistance bands

53 Cross-Body Shoulder Stretch
(Right, Left)

This sidearm stretch helps elongate the muscles in your back and arms and keeps them flexible.

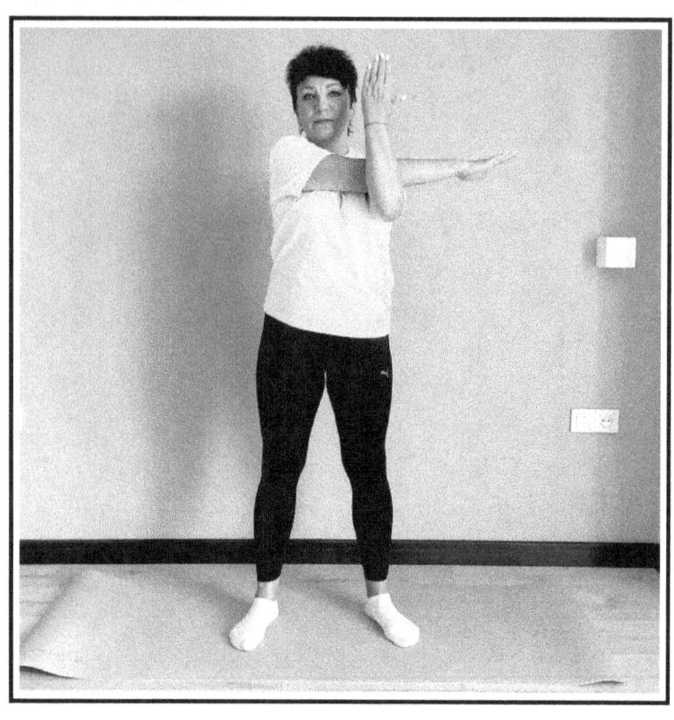 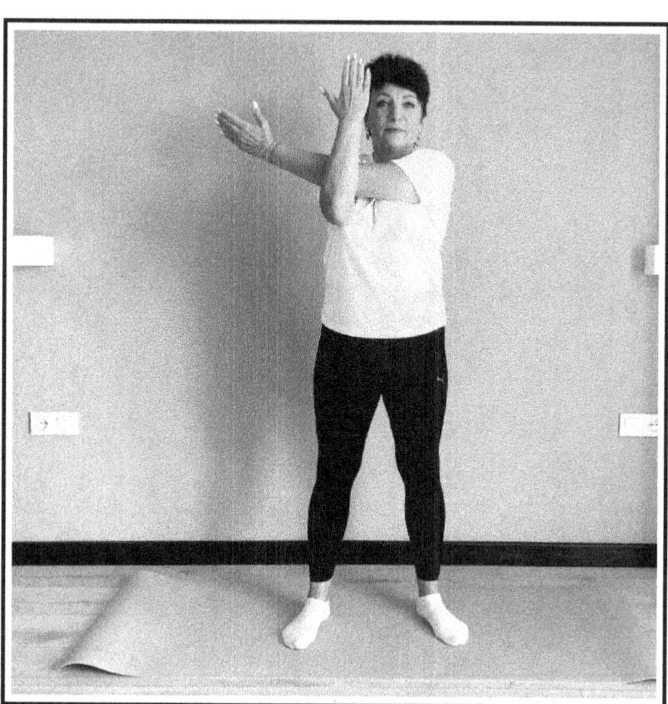

1. Stand or sit tall while grabbing one arm above your elbow with your opposite hand; pull it across your body toward your chest until you feel a stretch in your shoulder
2. Keep your elbow below shoulder height
3. Hold the stretch
4. Perform the exercise on the other side

- Don't lift your shoulder to the ear
- Don't bend your elbow while stretching your shoulder
- While stretching, breathe deep to help the muscles relax

Hamstring Stretch with a Band (Right, Left)

This exercise will give you a phenomenal stretch in your hamstrings and calves.

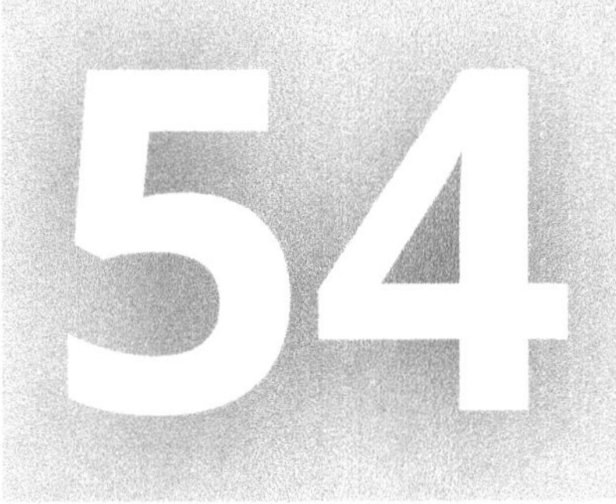

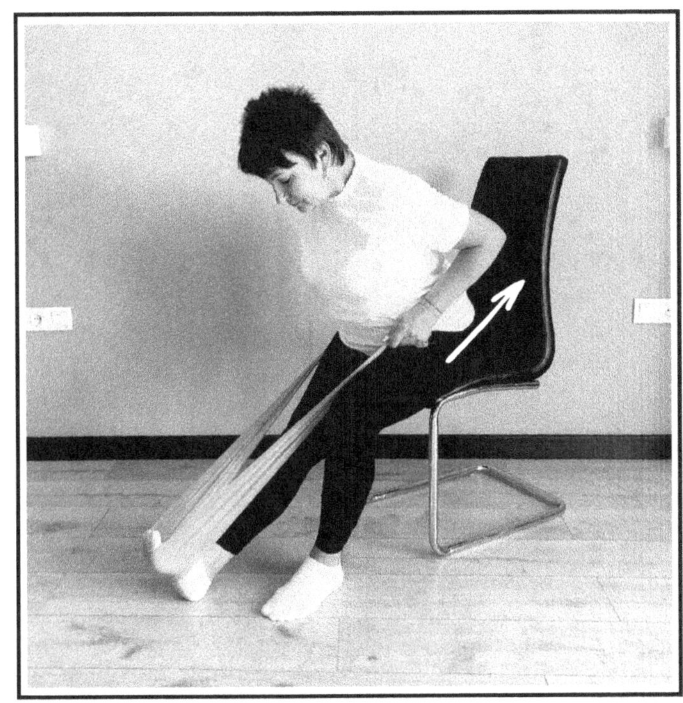

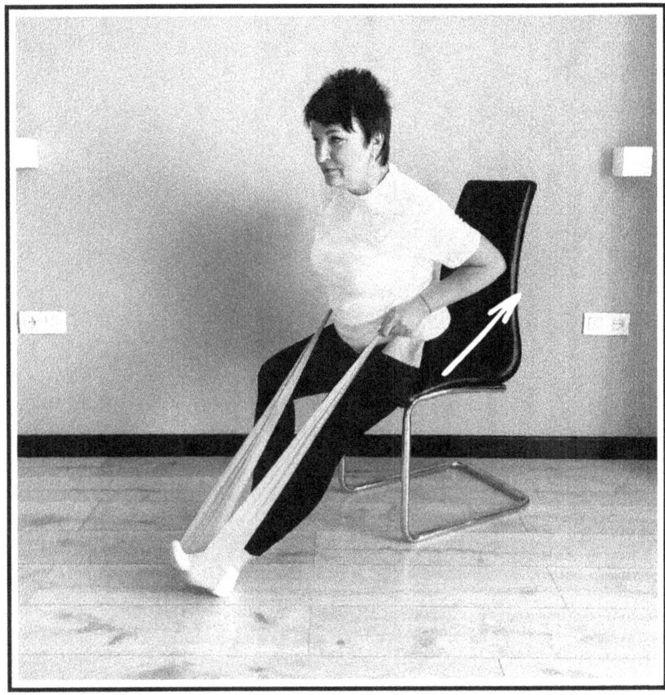

PROCEDURE:

1. Sit tall on a chair while extending your right foot forward
2. Loop the band under your right toes
3. Stretch the band and lean forward slowly toward the right leg
4. Hold the static position
5. Perform the exercise using the left leg

SUGGESTED TIPS:

- Don't rush the movement
- Don't arch the back
- At the beginning of the movement, inhale; as you lean forward, slowly exhale

Standing Quad Stretch
(Right, Left)

This simple stretch exercise is great for warming up your muscles anytime and anywhere.

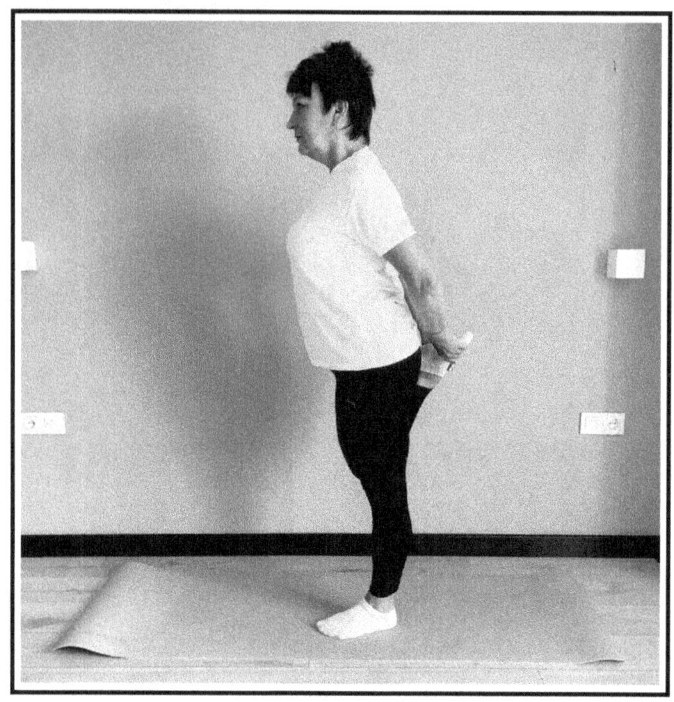 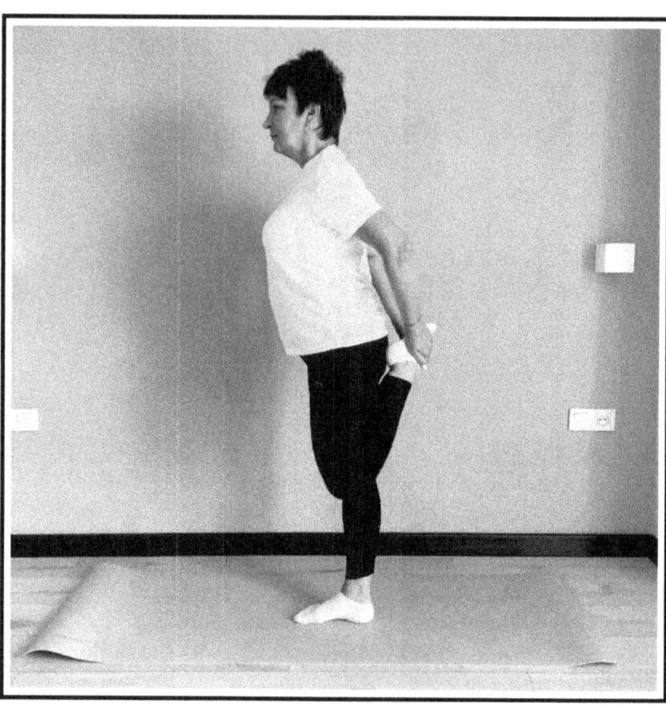

PROCEDURE:

1. Stand on your left leg with your knees together
2. Grab your right foot with your right hand; pull it toward your butt
3. Hold the stretch
4. Perform the exercise using the left foot

SUGGESTED TIPS:

- Don't lean forward with your back
- Keep your knees together
- Hold onto a chair or lean slightly on the wall to keep you steady if needed
- Push your chest up and hips forward to get a good hip flexor stretch and feel the stretch in the quad muscle

Overhead Lat Stretch
(Right, Left)

This relaxing stretch helps relieve tension in the triceps and lower shoulder.

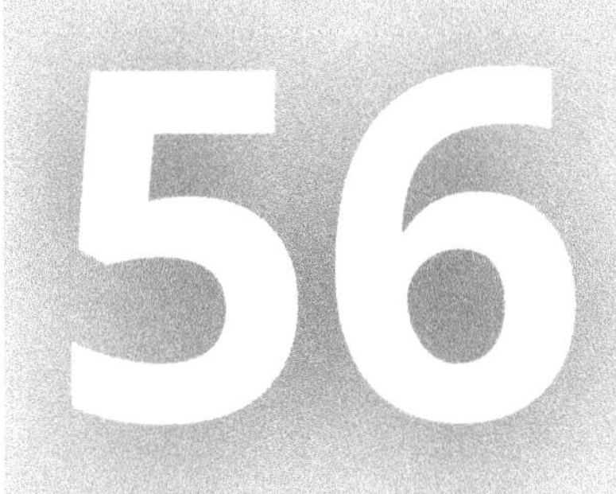

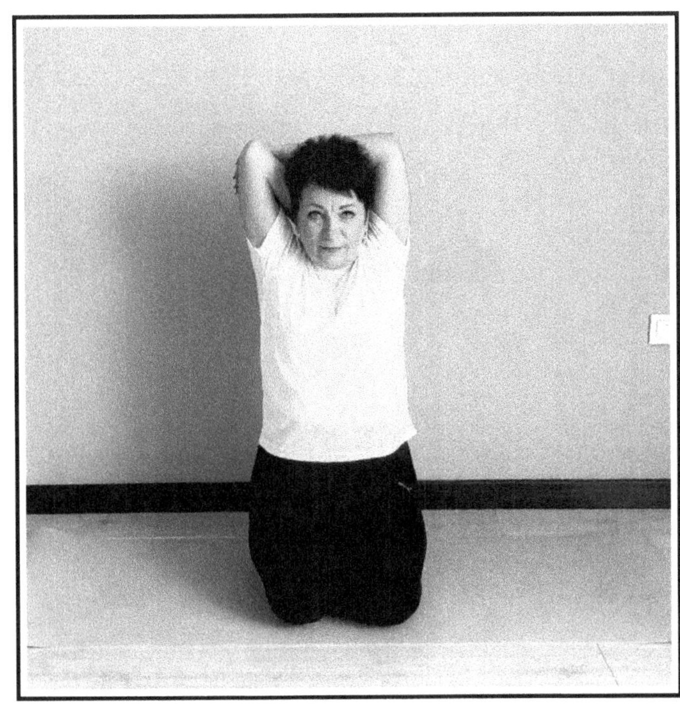

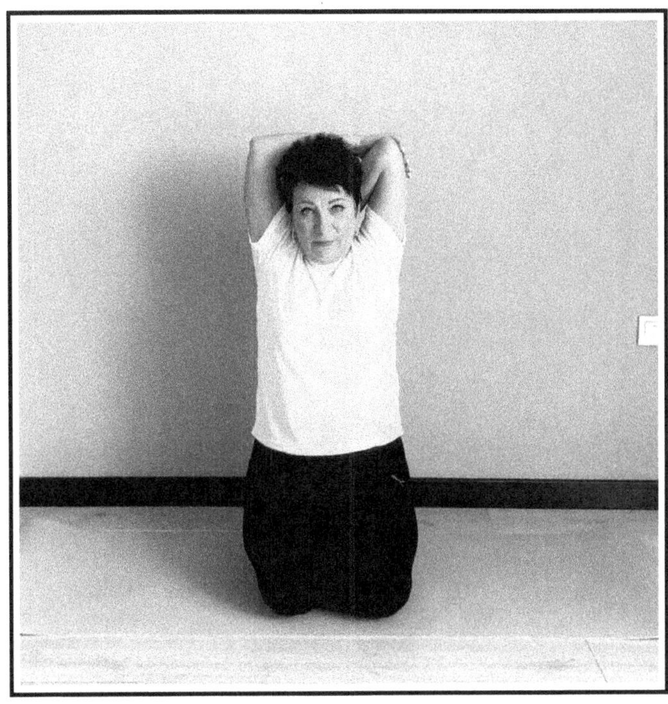

PROCEDURE:

1. Stand or sit tall while extending your right arm above the head
2. Bend the elbow and reach your hand between the shoulder blades
3. Grab the right elbow with your left hand and pull it toward the midline of your body
4. Hold the stretch
5. Perform the same exercise on the other side

SUGGESTED TIPS:

- Don't flex the triceps too much
- Keep the arm relaxed for the best stretch
- Breathe deeply throughout the stretch to relax your body
- If it is uncomfortable to sit, perform the exercise standing

57 Seated Lower Back Stretch
(Right, Left)

This is one of the best exercises to loosen your lower back.

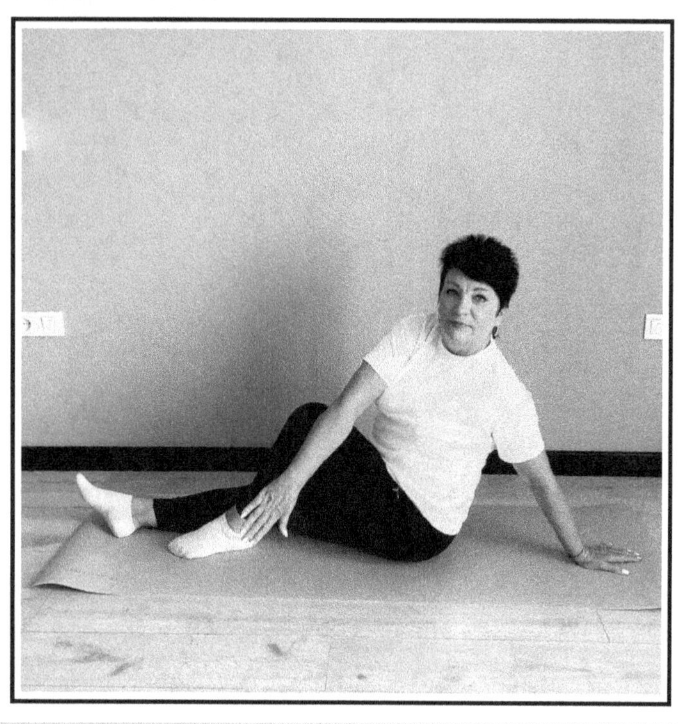 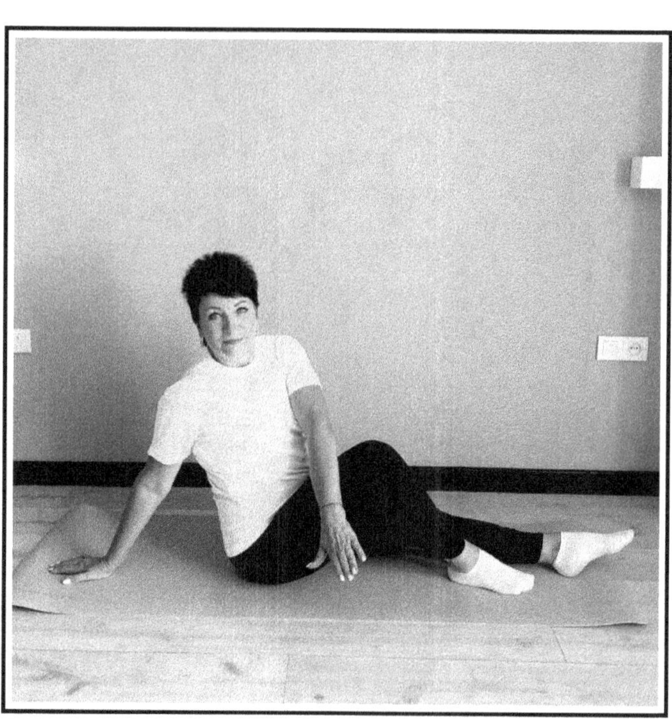

PROCEDURE:

1. Sit on the floor; bend your left leg, placing your foot flat on the floor
2. Reach your right arm across your left knee and place your left hand on the floor behind your body for balance
3. Push against your knee to twist the torso
4. Hold the stretch
5. Perform the exercise using the right foot over the left knee

SUGGESTED TIPS:

- Sit upright to stretch your lower back (don't slouch)
- Before starting the stretch, take a deep breath; as you stretch, exhale fully

Side Stretch (Right, Left)

This exercise stretches your abs and your thighs.

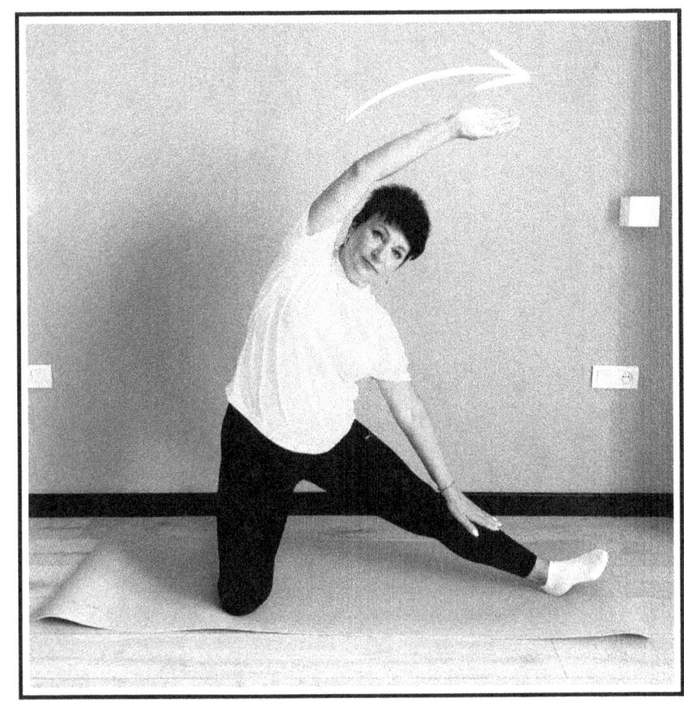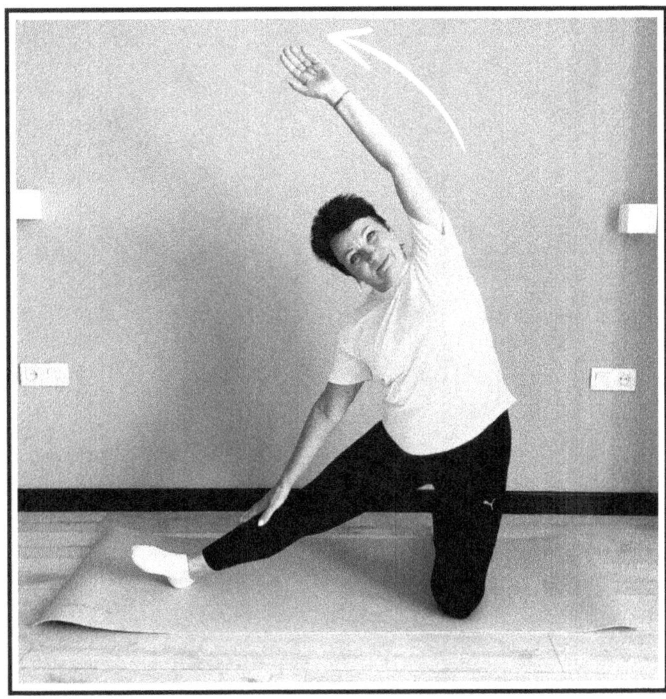

1. Kneel on the floor; straighten your left leg out to the side
2. Reach above your head with your right arm and let it lead your torso to bend toward your left leg
3. Hold the stretch
4. Perform the same exercise on the other side

- Don't bend your back forward or backward; try to stay steady while leaning to the side
- Feeling a stretch in your right thigh is a bonus (try pushing your left hip out to the side if you don't feel a stretch in the obliques and for a tougher stretch)

Sphinx Pose

This a great Pilates exercise to target your triceps, shoulders, lower back, chest, and abs.

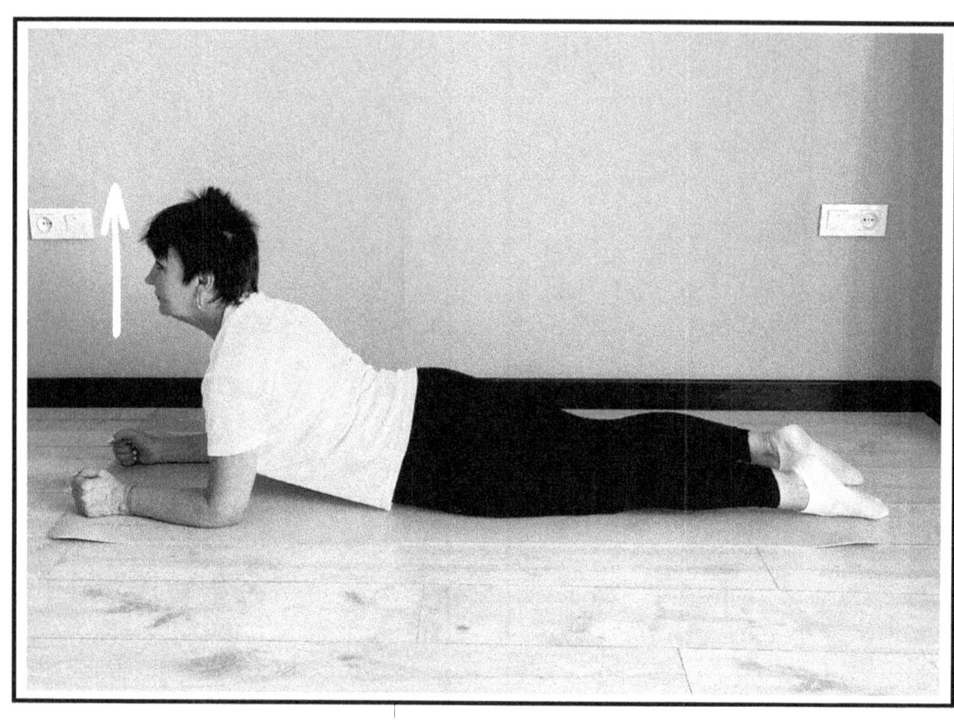

PROCEDURE:

1. Lie face down on the mat while resting on your forearms
2. Press your elbows down against the floor
3. Lift your chest and head slowly using your back muscles
4. Gently arch your back; hold the stretch

SUGGESTED TIPS:

- Don't overextend the neck
- Make sure to lift the chest off the floor
- Don't jam your shoulders toward your ears
- Avoid this pose if you have an injured lower back
- If you feel any pain throughout the exercise, stop and slowly lower yourself back down

PAGE 80

Cat to Cow Stretch

The cat exercise in Pilates is one of the simplest and gentlest ways to stretch out the back.

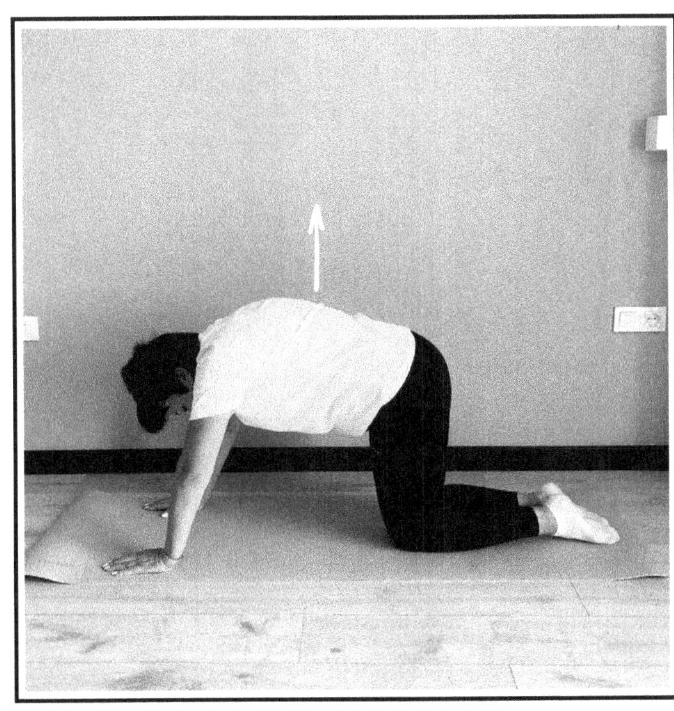 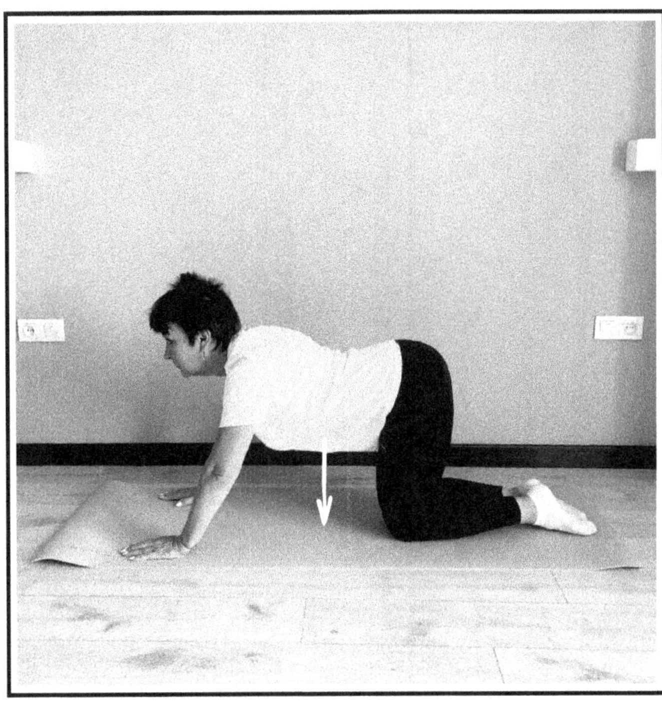

1. Get on all fours; place your hands directly under the shoulders and your knees under the hips
2. Inhale: Arch your back slightly and allow your head to rise and your butt to stick up and out
3. Exhale: Pull your navel in toward your spine and squeeze your butt low; repeat

- While arching your back, keep your rib cage and abdominals pulled in
- Don't strain the neck
- Keep the arms straight so the movement is with the spine (not with your arms and elbows)

61 Seated Forward Fold

The Seated Forward Fold exercise stretches the calves and hamstring muscles and mobilizes the lower and upper back.

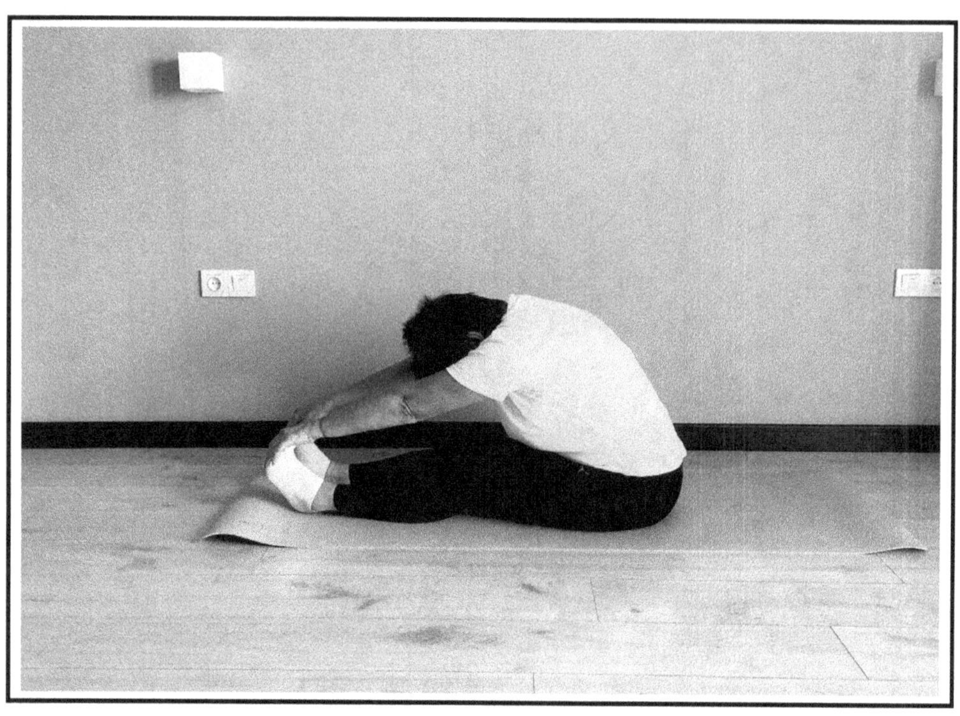

PROCEDURE:

1. Sit up tall
2. Keep the legs extended and bring together
3. Bend the body forward until you can touch the ankles with the fingers
4. Hold the static stretch

SUGGESTED TIPS:

- Use the full range of movement (unless you are lacking flexibility in hamstrings or lower back – then reduce the range of motion)
- Don't bend the arms or legs
- Continue breathing throughout the exercise

Child's Pose

The Child's Pose exercise can help relieve back pain and gently stretch the thighs, hips, back, and ankles.

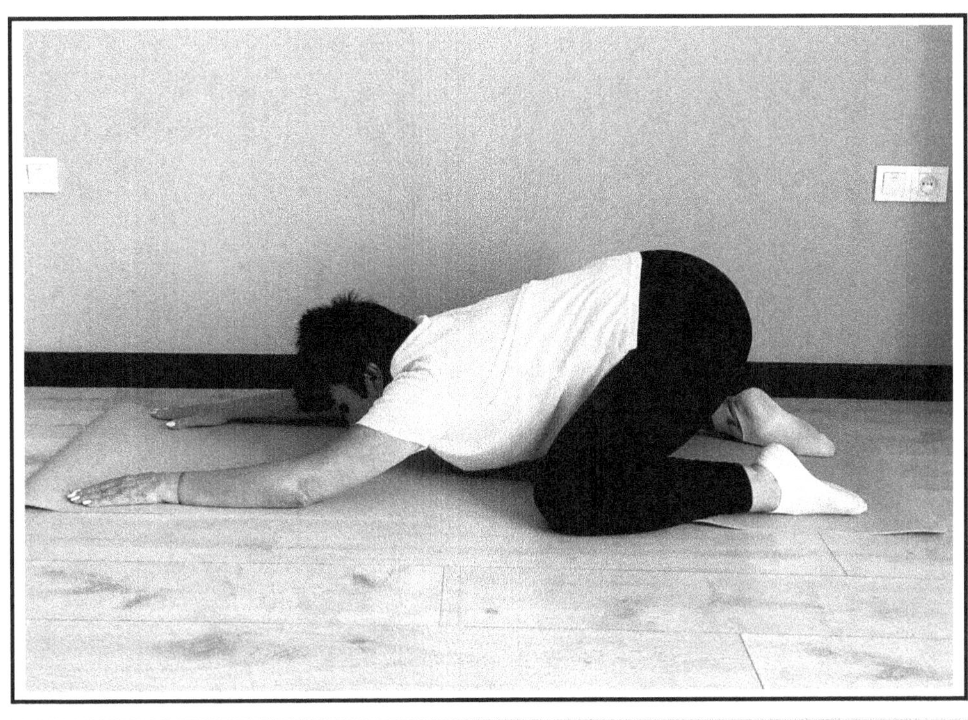

PROCEDURE:

1. Spread the knees wide, keeping the tops of your feet on the floor with the big toes touching
2. Bring the belly to rest on the floor between the forehead and thighs
3. Either stretch the arms in front of you with palms toward the floor or bring the arms back alongside your thighs with the palms facing upward
4. Remain in the position as long as you like; reconnect with the steady inhale of your breathing

SUGGESTED TIPS:

- Don't bend the neck; keep in a neutral position (use a pillow if needed)
- Avoid the exercise if you have a knee injury. Keep the arms by the side to provide support if you have a shoulder injury.

Static Lateral Lunge
(Right, Left)

This static stretch helps loosen up the side muscles and improves your flexibility.

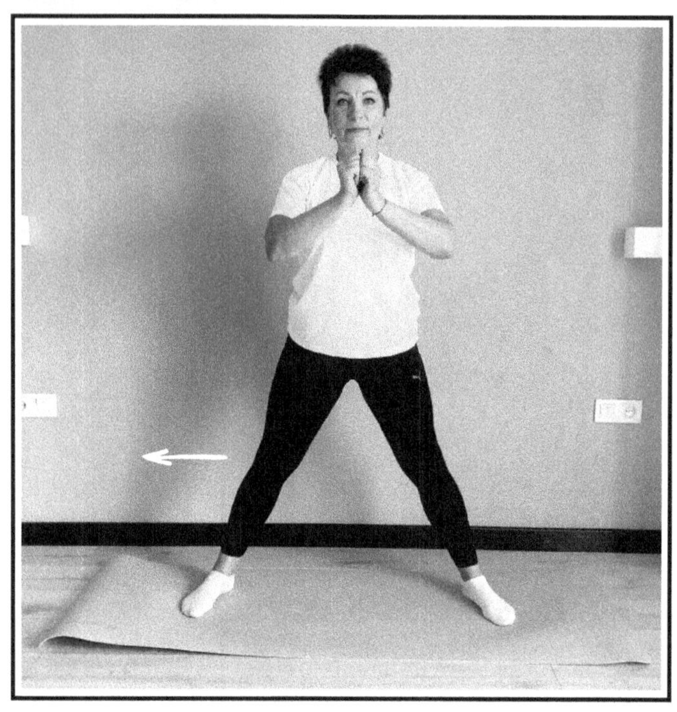

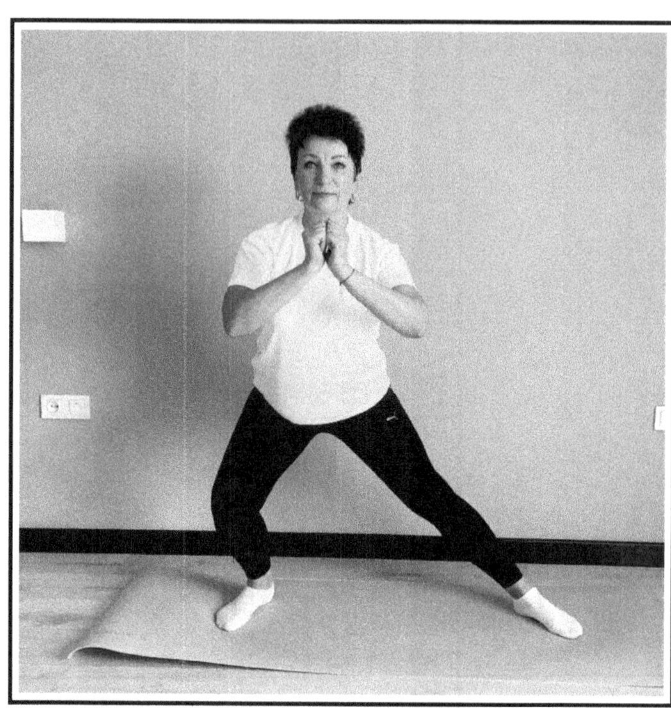

PROCEDURE:

1. Stand with your feet wider than shoulder-width apart; have a straight back with your weight on the heels
2. Drop the hips down and back; your right leg should be bent (around 90 degrees)
3. Keep the left leg straight
4. Hold the stretch
5. Perform the exercise on the other side

SUGGESTED TIPS:

- The bent knee should not go past your toes
- Don't hunch the back
- Make sure to keep your weight on your heels
- Engage the core
- Keep both soles of the feet on the floor as you lower

Cross-Legged Chest to Floor

This is a perfect stretching exercise for your piriformis muscles, hamstrings, and glutes. It stretches and elongates the spine, too.

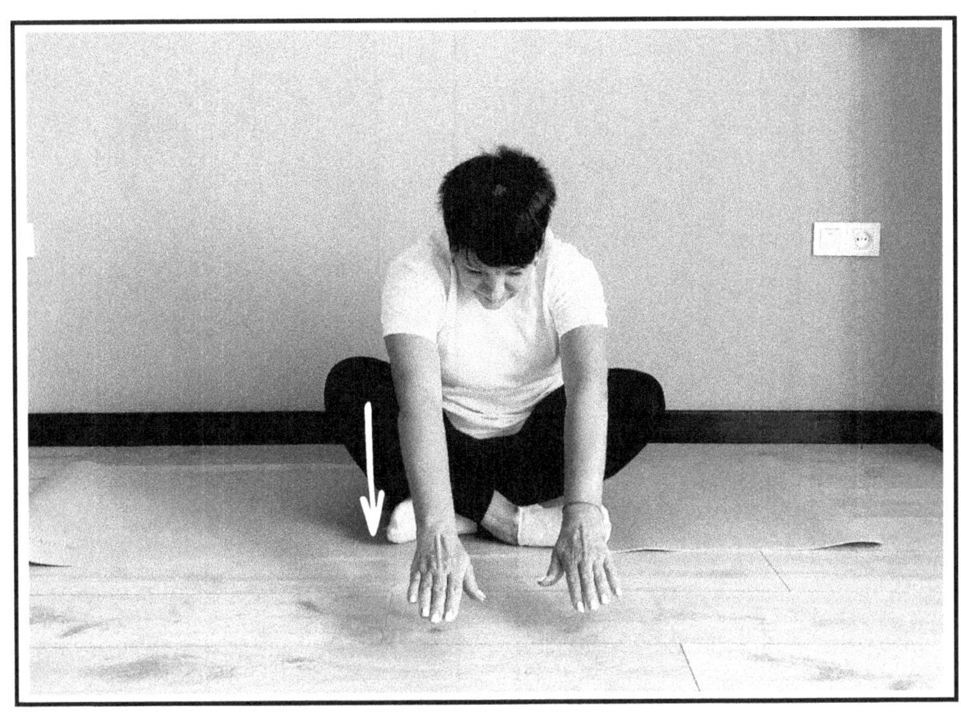

PROCEDURE:

1. Sit cross-legged; arms to the side
2. Reach to the ceiling with your arms
3. Bend from your hips and lower the body down drawing your navel into the lower back
4. Reach with your arms as far as comfortable, letting the chest hover over the legs
5. Hold this position

SUGGESTED TIPS:

- Move slowly; don't lower too far if the muscles aren't ready or if you feel pain

Hip Flexor Stretch
(Right, Left)

This common stretch is great for loosening up tight hips.

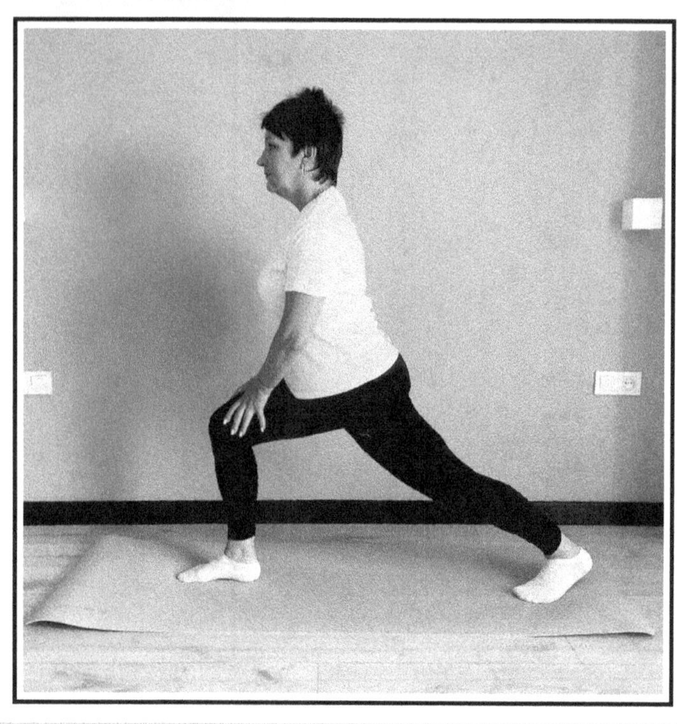
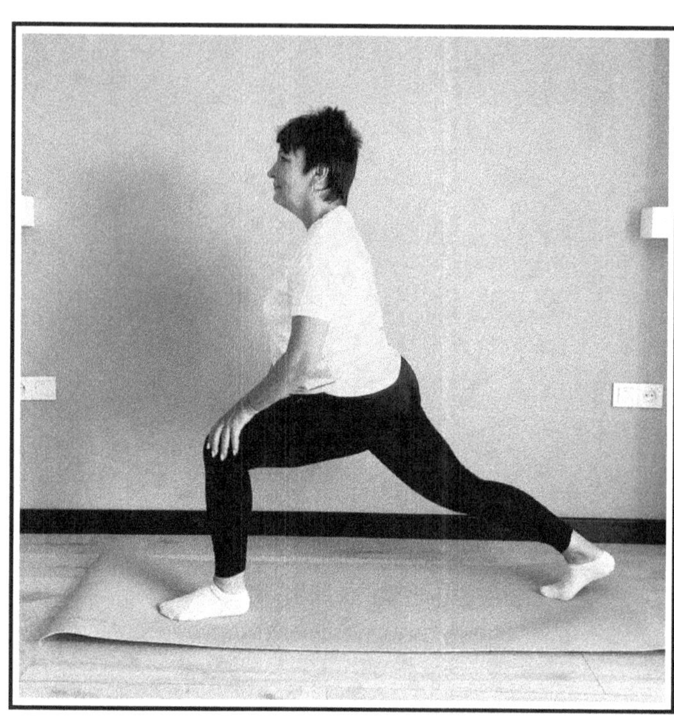

PROCEDURE:

1. Place the right knee on the floor behind you; your left leg bent at a 90-degree angle in front of you
2. Lean forward into your left knee; straighten and stretch your right hip flexor
3. Hold the position
4. Perform the exercise using the other leg

SUGGESTED TIPS:

- Keep your left knee behind the left toes
- If it's difficult to get the right leg straight, bring the right knee under the right hip and start from this position, lean forward until you feel a stretch; then slowly work the knee further back as needed

Figure 4 Stretch
(Right, Left)

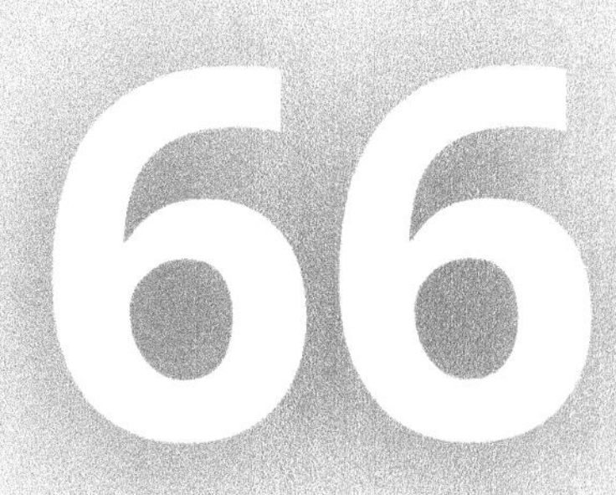

This is an all-around hip cradle stretch to loosen the hamstrings and glutes.

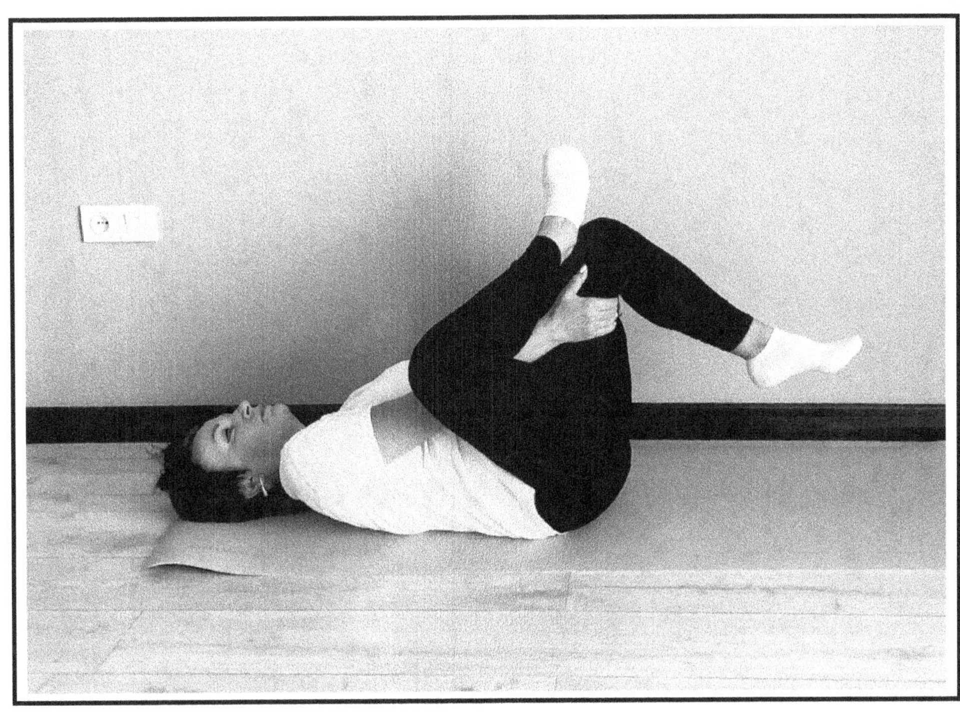

1. Lie on your back, bringing your left knee up so that your left foot is flat on the floor
2. Raise your right leg and rest your right calf right above the knee on your left quad
3. Reach under your left knee; pull both legs off the floor toward you; hold the stretch
4. Perform the exercise using the other leg

- Pull your chest up to meet your legs
- Try to stay relaxed and keep your back flat on the floor
- Once in position, breathe deeply, let your body relax, and stretch naturally

67 Standing Single Leg Forward Stretch (Right, Left)

This exercise promotes lower body flexibility, improves balance, and relieves tight hamstrings.

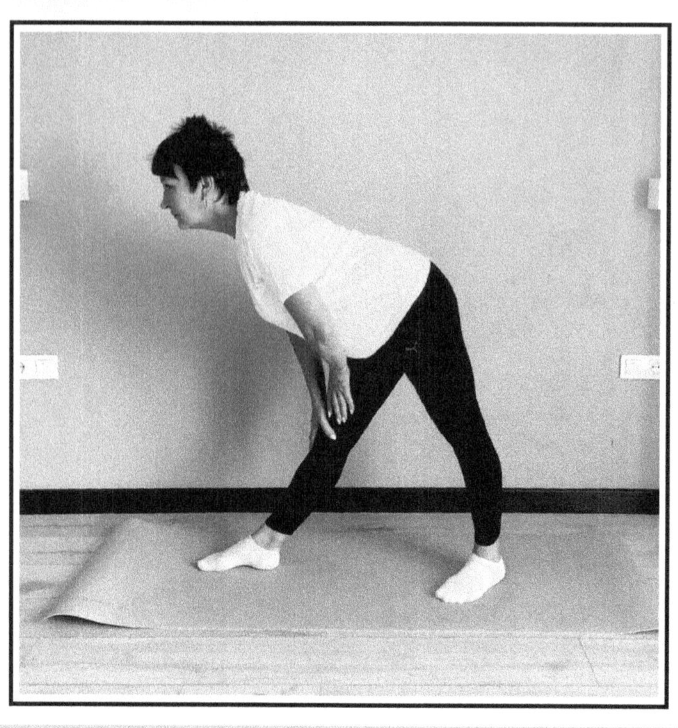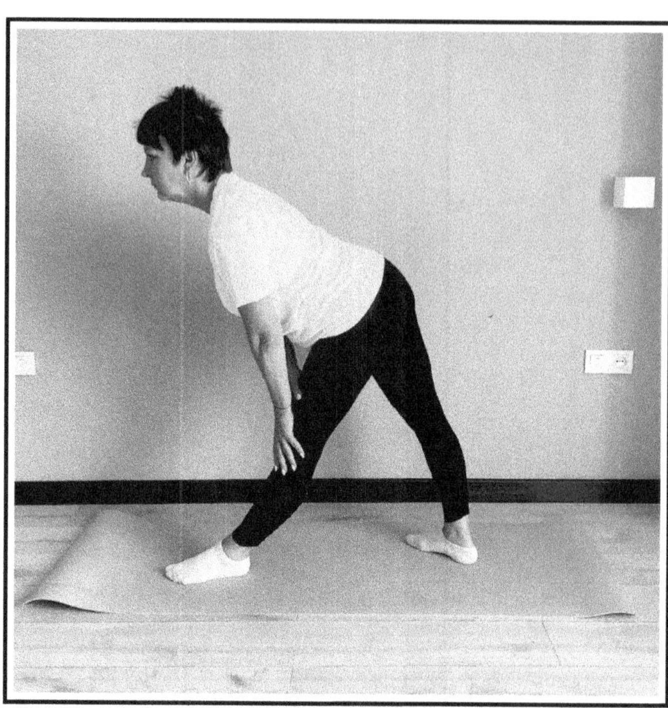

PROCEDURE:

1. Start in a right lunge
2. Lift your hips and lengthen both legs
3. Place your hands on the right leg
4. Turn your back heel down; your foot should be at a 45-degree angle with the hips squared
5. Hold this position
6. Perform the exercise using the other leg

SUGGESTED TIPS:

- Keep your knees straight
- Lengthen the torso forward
- Don't round your back
- Place the center of your right kneecap in line with the center of the right ankle

Standing Cross-Legged Forward Fold (Right, Left)

This exercise stretches the lateral hamstrings and targets the erector spinal muscles.

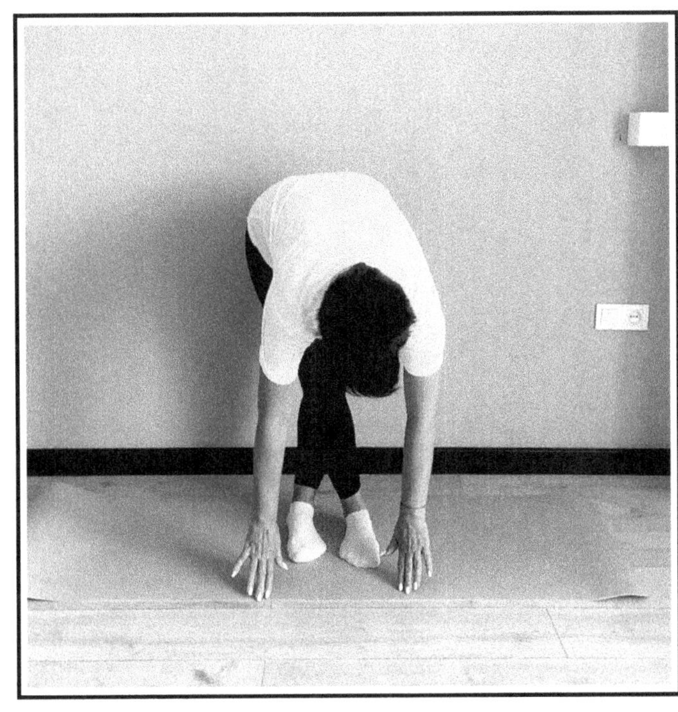

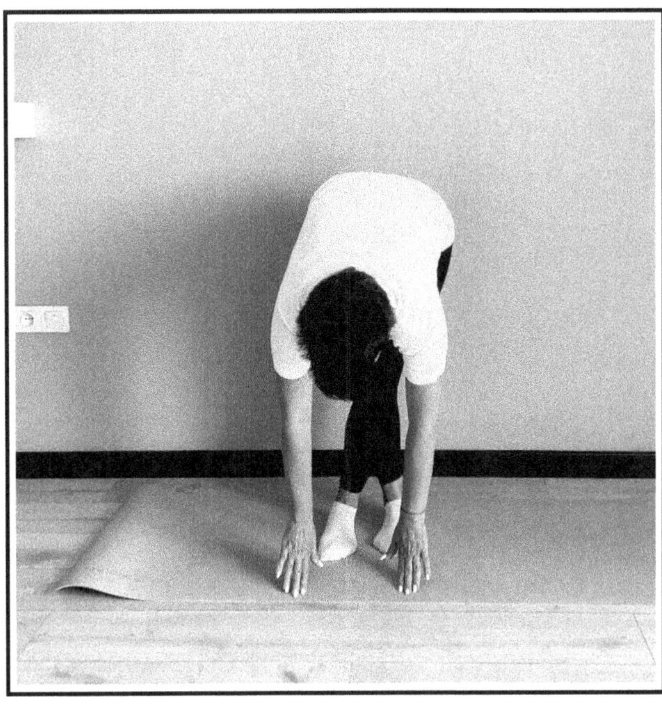

PROCEDURE:

1. Cross your right leg over the left leg
2. Lower your upper body into a forward fold
3. Place the hands on the floor
4. Gently press the chest toward your knees
5. Hold this position
6. Perform the same exercise by crossing your left leg over the right leg

SUGGESTED TIPS:

- Don't tense up the neck
- Lengthen the spine
- Equalize the weight between the feet; extend through the legs to get a stretch (if your hamstrings are too tight, bend the knees slightly so as not to pull or tear any muscles)

Knee to Chest Stretch
(Right, Left)

This is a relaxing stretch that opens your hips and relieves tension in the lower back.

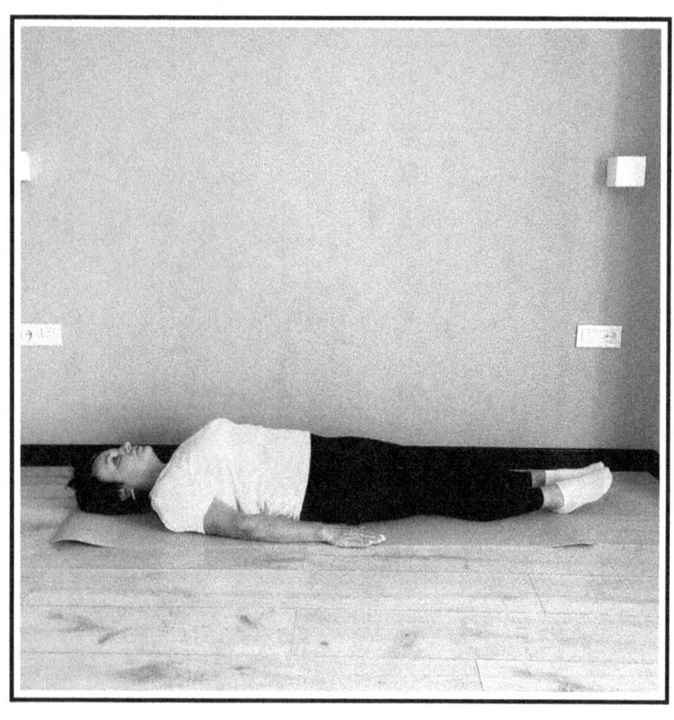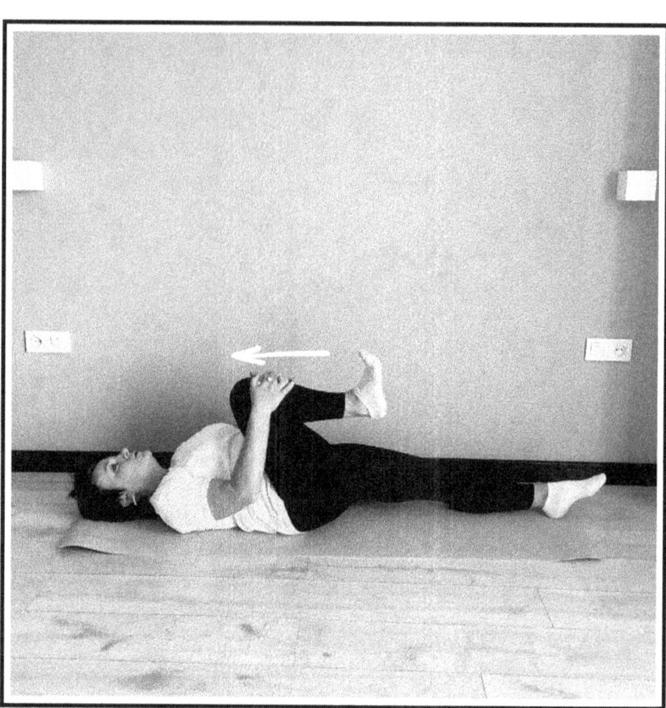

PROCEDURE:

1. Lie on the floor with legs stretched out
2. Bring your left knee up toward your chest; hug the knee into your torso with the arms
3. Hold the position
4. Perform the exercise with the other knee

SUGGESTED TIPS:

- Keep the back flat
- If it's difficult to hug the knee, hold a towel in your hands and pull it toward you (you will be able to do a full knee hug through continued practice)

Frog Stretch

70

The Frog Stretch works on adductor flexibility.

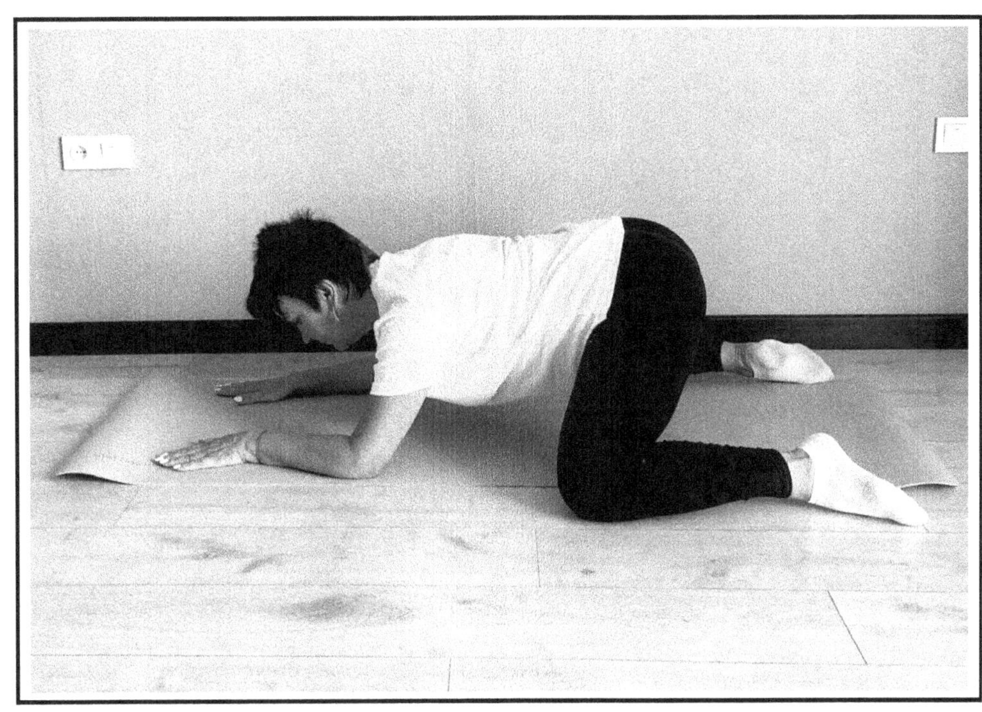

PROCEDURE:

1. Lie on your stomach
2. Rest on the elbows and knees
3. Open knees as wide as possible
4. Hold the static position

SUGGESTED TIPS:

- Don't arch the lower back
- Continue to breathe throughout the exercise (maintain a steady breathing pattern)

28-Day Workout Challenge

DAY 1

Upper Body

WARM-UP
1 - 30/30 sec
2 - 30/30 sec
8 - 30 sec

MAIN WORKOUT
26 - 40 sec
28 - 40 sec
17 - 40 sec
24 - 40/40 sec
31 - 40 sec

STRETCHING
53 - 30/30 sec
58 - 30/30 sec
61 - 30 sec

DAY 2

Full Body

WARM-UP
3 - 30/30 sec
13 - 30 sec
9 - 30 sec

MAIN WORKOUT
28 - 40 sec
20 - 40 sec
18 - 40 sec
47 - 40/40 sec
36 - 40/40 sec

STRETCHING
52 - 30/30 sec
69 - 30/30 sec
59 - 30 sec

DAY 3

Lower Body

WARM-UP
16 - 30 sec
6 - 30/30 sec
14 - 30/30 sec

MAIN WORKOUT
33 - 40 sec
32 - 40/40 sec
36 - 40/40 sec
39 - 40/40 sec
40 - 40 sec

STRETCHING
54 - 30 sec
67 - 30/30 sec
57 - 30/30 sec

DAY 4

Full Body

WARM-UP
11 - 30 sec
12 - 30 sec
5 - 30/30 sec

MAIN WORKOUT
17 - 40 sec
18 - 40 sec
49 - 40 sec
38 - 40/40 sec
42 - 40/40 sec

STRETCHING
58 - 30/30 sec
55 - 30/30 sec
62 - 30 sec

DAY 5

Upper Body

WARM-UP
4 - 30/30 sec
7 - 30 sec
10 - 30 sec

MAIN WORKOUT
19 - 40 sec
29 - 40/40 sec
30 - 40/40 sec
23 - 40 sec
27 - 40 sec

STRETCHING
52 - 30/30 sec
56 - 30/30 sec
60 - 30 sec

DAY 6

Full Body

WARM-UP
2 - 30/30 sec
15 - 30 sec
13 - 30 sec

MAIN WORKOUT
21 - 40 sec
26 - 40 sec
23 - 40 sec
39 - 40/40 sec
40 - 40 sec

STRETCHING
63 - 30/30 sec
66 - 30/30 sec
64 - 30 sec

Take a 15-30 second break between exercises, depending on how you feel, to allow your body to recover and maintain optimal performance

DAY 7

DAY OFF

DAY 8

Lower Body

WARM-UP
14 - 30/30 sec
10 - 30 sec
6 - 30/30 sec

MAIN WORKOUT
34 - 40/40 sec
45 - 40/40 sec
46 - 40 sec
48 - 40 sec
43 - 40 sec

STRETCHING
54 - 30 sec
68 - 30/30 sec
70 - 30 sec

DAY 9

Full Body

WARM-UP
3 - 30/30 sec
12 - 30 sec
5 - 30/30 sec

MAIN WORKOUT
26 - 40 sec
50 - 40 sec
44 - 40/40 sec
45 - 40/40 sec
27 - 40 sec

STRETCHING
58 - 30/30 sec
54 - 30 sec
60 - 30 sec

DAY 10

Upper Body

WARM-UP
1 - 30/30 sec
2 - 30/30 sec
8 - 30 sec

MAIN WORKOUT
21 - 40 sec
25 - 40 sec
28 - 40 sec
29 - 40/40 sec
30 - 40/40 sec

STRETCHING
53 - 30/30 sec
58 - 30/30 sec
61 - 30 sec

DAY 11

Full Body

WARM-UP
3 - 30/30 sec
13 - 30 sec
9 - 30 sec

MAIN WORKOUT
19 - 40 sec
20 - 40 sec
46 - 40 sec
47 - 40/40 sec
37 - 40/40 sec

STRETCHING
52 - 30/30 sec
69 - 30/30 sec
59 - 30 sec

DAY 12

Lower Body

WARM-UP
16 - 30 sec
6 - 30/30 sec
14 - 30/30 sec

MAIN WORKOUT
41 - 40/40 sec
50 - 40 sec
48 - 40 sec
51 - 40 sec
43 - 40 sec

STRETCHING
54 - 30 sec
67 - 30/30 sec
57 - 30/30 sec

DAY 13

Full Body

WARM-UP
11 - 30 sec
12 - 30 sec
5 - 30/30 sec

MAIN WORKOUT
49 - 40 sec
25 - 40 sec
31 - 40 sec
44 - 40/40 sec
37 - 40/40 sec

STRETCHING
58 - 30/30 sec
55 - 30/30 sec
62 - 30 sec

Take a 15-30 second break between exercises, depending on how you feel, to allow your body to recover and maintain optimal performance

DAY 14

DAY OFF

DAY 15
Upper Body

WARM-UP
4 - 30/30 sec
7 - 30 sec
10 - 30 sec

MAIN WORKOUT
26 - 40 sec
28 - 40 sec
17 - 40 sec
24 - 40/40 sec
31 - 40 sec
29 - 40/40 sec

STRETCHING
52 - 30/30 sec
56 - 30/30 sec
60 - 30 sec

DAY 16
Full Body

WARM-UP
2 - 30/30 sec
15 - 30 sec
13 - 30 sec

MAIN WORKOUT
28 - 40 sec
20 - 40 sec
18 - 40 sec
47 - 40/40 sec
36 - 40/40 sec
32 - 40/40 sec

STRETCHING
63 - 30/30 sec
66 - 30/30 sec
64 - 30 sec

DAY 17
Lower Body

WARM-UP
14 - 30/30 sec
10 - 30 sec
6 - 30/30 sec

MAIN WORKOUT
33 - 40 sec
32 - 40/40 sec
36 - 40/40 sec
39 - 40/40 sec
40 - 40 sec
26 - 40 sec

STRETCHING
54 - 30 sec
68 - 30/30 sec
70 - 30 sec

DAY 18
Full Body

WARM-UP
3 - 30/30 sec
12 - 30 sec
5 - 30/30 sec

MAIN WORKOUT
17 - 40 sec
18 - 40 sec
49 - 40 sec
38 - 40/40 sec
42 - 40/40 sec
51 - 40 sec

STRETCHING
58 - 30/30 sec
54 - 30 sec
60 - 30 sec

DAY 19
Upper Body

WARM-UP
1 - 30/30 sec
2 - 30/30 sec
8 - 30 sec

MAIN WORKOUT
19 - 40 sec
29 - 40/40 sec
30 - 40/40 sec
23 - 40 sec
27 - 40 sec
41 - 40/40 sec

STRETCHING
53 - 30/30 sec
58 - 30/30 sec
61 - 30 sec

DAY 20
Full Body

WARM-UP
3 - 30/30 sec
13 - 30 sec
9 - 30 sec

MAIN WORKOUT
21 - 40 sec
26 - 40 sec
23 - 40 sec
39 - 40/40 sec
40 - 40 sec
35 - 40/40 sec

STRETCHING
52 - 30/30 sec
69 - 30/30 sec
59 - 30 sec

Take a 15-30 second break between exercises, depending on how you feel, to allow your body to recover and maintain optimal performance

DAY 21
DAY OFF

DAY 22
Lower Body

WARM-UP
16 - 30 sec
6 - 30/30 sec
14 - 30/30 sec

MAIN WORKOUT
34 - 50/50 sec
45 - 50/50 sec
46 - 50 sec
48 - 50 sec
43 - 50 sec
42 - 50/50 sec

STRETCHING
54 - 30 sec
67 - 30/30 sec
57 - 30/30 sec

DAY 23
Full Body

WARM-UP
11 - 30 sec
12 - 30 sec
5 - 30/30 sec

MAIN WORKOUT
26 - 50 sec
50 - 50 sec
44 - 50/50 sec
45 - 50/50 sec
27 - 50 sec
34 - 50/50 sec

STRETCHING
58 - 30/30 sec
55 - 30/30 sec
62 - 30 sec

DAY 24
Upper Body

WARM-UP
4 - 30/30 sec
7 - 30 sec
10 - 30 sec

MAIN WORKOUT
21 - 50 sec
25 - 50 sec
28 - 50 sec
29 - 50/50 sec
30 - 50/50 sec
22 - 50 sec

STRETCHING
52 - 30/30 sec
56 - 30/30 sec
60 - 30 sec

DAY 25
Full Body

WARM-UP
2 - 30/30 sec
15 - 30 sec
13 - 30 sec

MAIN WORKOUT
19 - 50 sec
20 - 50 sec
46 - 50 sec
47 - 50/50 sec
37 - 50/50 sec
28 - 50 sec

STRETCHING
63 - 30/30 sec
66 - 30/30 sec
64 - 30 sec

DAY 26
Lower Body

WARM-UP
14 - 30/30 sec
10 - 30 sec
6 - 30/30 sec

MAIN WORKOUT
41 - 50/50 sec
50 - 50 sec
48 - 50 sec
51 - 50 sec
43 - 50 sec
24 - 50/50 sec

STRETCHING
54 - 30 sec
68 - 30/30 sec
70 - 30 sec

DAY 27
Full Body

WARM-UP
3 - 30/30 sec
12 - 30 sec
5 - 30/30 sec

MAIN WORKOUT
49 - 50 sec
25 - 50 sec
31 - 50 sec
44 - 50/50 sec
37 - 50/50 sec
30 - 50/50 sec

STRETCHING
58 - 30/30 sec
54 - 30 sec
60 - 30 sec

Take a 15-30 second break between exercises, depending on how you feel, to allow your body to recover and maintain optimal performance

DAY 28
DAY OFF

Conclusion

Congratulations on completing "Resistance Band Workout for Seniors". You've taken a significant step toward enhancing your health, strength, and overall well-being. Through the exercises and routines outlined in this book, you've discovered how simple resistance bands can transform your fitness journey, offering a safe, effective, and versatile way to stay active.

Remember, consistency is key. The benefits you've started to experience will continue to grow as you make resistance band workouts a regular part of your life. We encourage you to listen to your body, celebrate your progress, and challenge yourself with new goals. Embrace the joy of movement, the satisfaction of achieving your fitness milestones, and the vibrant energy of an active lifestyle.

Thank you for allowing us to be part of your fitness journey. Here's to a future filled with strength, health, and happiness. Stay active, stay vibrant, and continue to embrace the power of elastic vitality!

FitLife Solutions Team

References

- Resistance Band: Low Impact Workout Easy for Beginners. (n.d.). Better Me. https://betterme.world/

- Ayuda, Tiffany, Weg, Arielle, and Haase, Madeleine. (2024, May 14). 10 Best Resistance Band Leg Workouts to Tone Your Legs and Fire Up Your Glutes. Prevention. https://www.prevention.com/fitness/workouts/g29485708/resistance-band-exercises-for-legs/

- Fargo, Morgan and Wilkins, Bridie. (2024, June 20). 26 Best Resistance Band Exercises to Get Strong Without Weights. Women's Heath. https://www.womenshealthmag.com/uk/fitness/strength-training/a31986994/resistance-band-exercises/

- Team Peloton. (2023, May 17). 13 Amazing Resistance Band Exercises to Build Strength. Peloton the Output. https://www.onepeloton.com/blog/resistance-band-exercises/

- The Best Resistance Bands Exercises. (n.d.) bodylastics. https://bodylastics.com/resistance-bands-exercises/

ISBN: 9798333103253